Quality Measurement in Healthcare

Edited by

Jesse M. Pines

US Acute Care Solutions, Canton, OH, USA

Department of Emergency Medicine, School of Medicine and Health Sciences, The George Washington University, Washington, DC, USA

Helen Burstin

Council of Medical Specialty Societies (CMSS), Washington, DC, USA

Department of Medicine, School of Medicine and Health Sciences, The George Washington University, Washington, DC, USA

Jane Hyatt Thorpe

Department of Health Policy and Management, Milken Institute School of Public Health, The George Washington University, Washington, DC, USA

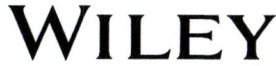

Registered Office(s)
John Wiley & Sons, Inc., 111 River Street, Hoboken, NJ 07030, USA
John Wiley & Sons Ltd, New Era House, 8 Oldlands Way, Bognor Regis, West Sussex, PO22 9NQ, UK

For details of our global editorial offices, customer services, and more information about Wiley products visit us at www.wiley.com.

The manufacturer's authorized representative according to the EU General Product Safety Regulation is Wiley-VCH GmbH, Boschstr. 12, 69469 Weinheim, Germany, e-mail: Product_Safety@wiley.com.

Library of Congress Cataloging-in-Publication Data Applied for:

Paperback ISBN: 9781394219391

Cover Design: Wiley
Cover Image: © elenabsl/stock.adobe.com

Set in 11.5/13.5pts STIXTwoText by Straive, Pondicherry, India

To my children, Asher, Molly, and Oren, and my wife, Lori, who remind me every day of the importance of care, compassion, and striving for the best in all we do.

—Jesse M. Pines

Dedicated to Mark, Deena, and Sam for their unwavering support for my work and to the healthcare professionals who tirelessly work to ensure that all patients receive the best possible care.

—Helen Burstin

To my parents, Bill and Judy Thorpe; my husband, Michael Sramek; and our daughters, Carolina and Virginia, who inspire and encourage me in their own special ways.

To my students at The George Washington University, Milken Institute School of Public Health, who will carry this important work forward and continue to improve healthcare access, quality, equity, and affordability.

—Jane Hyatt Thorpe

Contents

7 Patient Safety Measurement 91

Edward J. Septimus

8 Patient-Reported Outcomes in Performance Measures 107

Margaret Morris, Patricia D. Franklin, Nan E. Rothrock, and David Cella

*Jill A. Marsteller, Christina A. Vincent, Andrew Anderson, John Jackson,
J. Matthew Austin, and Lisa A. Cooper*

List of Contributors

Taroon Amin
Independent Consultant
New York, NY
USA

Andrew Anderson
Department of Health Policy and
Management
Johns Hopkins Bloomberg School
of Public Health
Baltimore, MD
USA

Heidi Bossley
Bossley Consulting, LLC
Alexandria, VA
USA

Helen Burstin
Council of Medical Specialty
Societies (CMSS)
Washington, DC
USA

and

Department of Medicine
School of Medicine and
Health Sciences
The George Washington University
Washington, DC
USA

David Cella
Department of Medical
Social Sciences
Northwestern University Feinberg
School of Medicine
Chicago, IL
USA

and

The Ken and Ruth Davee
Department of Neurology
Northwestern University
Feinberg School of Medicine
Chicago, IL
USA

and

Department of Psychiatry and
Behavioral Sciences
Northwestern University Feinberg
School of Medicine
Chicago, IL
USA

Candice Chen
The Fitzhugh Mullan Institute for
Health Workforce Equity
George Washington University
Milken Institute School of
Public Health
Washington, DC
USA

Lisa A. Cooper
Department of Medicine
Johns Hopkins Center for
Health Equity
Johns Hopkins School of Medicine
Baltimore, MD
USA

and

Department of Health,
Behavior and Society
Johns Hopkins Bloomberg School of
Public Health
Baltimore, MD
USA

and

Johns Hopkins School of Nursing
Baltimore, MD
USA

Karen S. Cosby
Department of Emergency Medicine
Rush University Medical Center
and Attending Physician
Cook County Health
Chicago, IL
USA

Monisha Dilip
Department of Emergency Medicine
Columbia University
New York, NY
USA

Lee A. Fleisher
University of Pennsylvania
Perelman School of Medicine
Duke Margolis Institute for
Health Policy
Durham, NC
USA

Patricia D. Franklin
Department of Medical
Social Sciences
Northwestern University Feinberg
School of Medicine
Chicago, IL
USA

and

Department of Orthopaedic Surgery
Northwestern University Feinberg
School of Medicine
Chicago, IL
USA

and

Department of Medicine
Northwestern University Feinberg
School of Medicine
Chicago, IL
USA

Jeffrey Geppert
Battelle
Columbus, OH
USA

Ashlie Wilbon Gyr
Booz Allen Hamilton
Atlanta, GA
USA

John Jackson
Department of Medicine
Johns Hopkins Center for
Health Equity
Johns Hopkins School of Medicine
Baltimore, MD
USA

and

Departments of Epidemiology
Mental Health, and Biostatistics
Johns Hopkins Bloomberg School
of Public Health
Baltimore, MD
USA

Karen Johnson
Quality & Measurement
American Urological Association
Linthicum Heights, MD
USA

Robert Lloyd
Improvement Science and Methods
Institute for Healthcare Improvement
Boston, MA
USA

Jill A. Marsteller
Department of Health Policy and
Management
Johns Hopkins Bloomberg School of
Public Health
Baltimore, MD
USA

and

Department of Medicine, Johns
Hopkins Center for Health Equity
Johns Hopkins School of Medicine
Baltimore, MD
USA

and

Armstrong Institute for Patient
Safety and Quality
Johns Hopkins School of Medicine
Baltimore, MD
USA

J. Matthew Austin
Armstrong Institute for Patient
Safety and Quality
Johns Hopkins School of Medicine
Baltimore, MD
USA

and

Department of Anesthesiology and
Critical Care Medicine
Johns Hopkins School of Medicine
Baltimore, MD
USA

Margaret Morris
Department of Medical Social Sciences
Northwestern University Feinberg
School of Medicine
Chicago, IL
USA

Jonathan B. Perlin
The Joint Commission/Joint
Commission International
USA

and

Vanderbilt University
Nashville, TN
USA

and

Virginia Commonwealth
University, Richmond, VA
USA

Jennifer Perloff
Institute for Healthcare Systems
Brandeis University
Waltham, MA
USA

Jesse M. Pines
US Acute Care Solutions
Canton, OH
USA

and

Department of Emergency Medicine
School of Medicine and
Health Sciences
The George Washington University
Washington, DC
USA

Brenna Rabel
Battelle
Columbus, OH
USA

Nan E. Rothrock
Department of Medical Social Sciences
Northwestern University Feinberg
School of Medicine
Chicago, IL
USA

and

The Ken and Ruth Davee
Department of Neurology
Northwestern University Feinberg
School of Medicine
Chicago, IL
USA

and

Department of Psychiatry and
Behavioral Sciences
Northwestern University Feinberg
School of Medicine
Chicago, IL
USA

Jeffrey Salvon-Harman
Safety, Institute for Healthcare
Improvement
Boston, MA
USA

Rohit B. Sangal
Yale Emergency Department
Yale School of Medicine
New Haven, CT
USA

Michelle Schreiber
Quality Measures and Value-Based
Incentive Group
Centers for Medicare and
Medicaid Services
Baltimore, MD
USA

Edward J. Septimus
Department of Population Medicine
Harvard Pilgrim Healthcare
Boston, MA
USA

Jane Hyatt Thorpe
Department of Health Policy and
Management
Milken Institute School of Public
Health, The George Washington
University
Washington, DC
USA

Arjun K. Venkatesh
Yale Emergency Department
Yale School of Medicine
New Haven, CT
USA

Christina A. Vincent
Department of Medicine
Johns Hopkins Center for
Health Equity
Johns Hopkins School of Medicine
Baltimore, MD
USA

Ian Warmbrodt
Battelle
Columbus, OH
USA

Preface

Healthcare Quality Measurement in the Twenty-First Century

High-quality healthcare is central to ensuring people receive effective, safe, and timely services and treatments and their health outcomes and well-being are optimized. "High quality" means care that aligns with the best evidence available, minimizes medical error risks, reduces preventable complications, and promotes equitable access to services. High-quality healthcare should also foster trust in the clinicians delivering care throughout the medical system. A trusting relationship between clinicians and patients encourages people to seek care when needed, adhere to prescribed treatments, and engage actively in their care and their health.

Quality measurement – the subject of this book – plays a critical role in moving the healthcare delivery enterprise toward the goal of high-quality healthcare. It does this by driving improvement in the form of actionable data by which organizations and individual clinicians can assess and enhance care delivery and, in doing so, improve patient outcomes. Quality measurement identifies care gaps, which guide the implementation of targeted interventions. It helps ensure accountability through close monitoring of progress over time. It also informs patients, clinicians, and policymakers about the quality and efficiency of healthcare delivery. Additionally, quality measurement facilitates the use of public reporting as well as value-based care models, where reimbursement is tied to patient outcomes rather than volume, incentivizing high-quality, patient-centered care.

This book gives readers a detailed tour through the definition, history, science, implementation, and future of quality measurement. As American authors and editors, we focus on how these services are deployed in the United States. However, many of the principles described in this book apply across the world, from other developed nations to emerging systems in less-developed countries. Importantly, this book is an assembly of the current thought leaders in the field. Many are the past and present architects of the current approaches to quality measurement and will continue to guide its future in the coming years.

The book has 15 chapters divided into four sections: (1) *What Is Quality and Why Should We Measure It in Healthcare?* (2) *How Do We Measure Quality in Healthcare?* (3) *How Do We Use Quality Measurement to Drive Change in Healthcare?* and (4) *How Might Quality Measurement In Healthcare Evolve?* Each chapter ends with a series of discussion questions that can be used to reflect on the content in the chapter and in didactic environments.

Our goal in publishing this book is to provide readers with the basics of what is needed to understand quality measurement. Ultimately, the practice of engaging in the quality measurement ecosystem, whether it be from the perspective of a clinician, an academic, a policymaker, a measure developer, an administrator, or a quality improvement professional, will offer a deeper knowledge into this highly technical field.

We – the editors – have dedicated a substantial part of our careers to the study, implementation, and teaching of quality measurement. We believe in the fundamental premise that by focusing on measurable aspects of care, healthcare systems and clinicians can strive for continuous improvement, fostering environments where excellence becomes the standard. Finally, this book represents a point in time in the history and current state of quality measurement. In the coming years, there will undoubtedly be advancements in the way that healthcare quality is assessed and quality improvement is implemented with new sources of data, new technology, and the ever-evolving policy landscape.

January 2025

Jesse M. Pines, MD, MBA

Helen Burstin, MD, MPH

Jane Hyatt Thorpe, JD

What Is Quality and Why Should We Measure It in Healthcare?

1 What Is Healthcare Quality Measurement?

Jane Hyatt Thorpe[1] and Jesse M. Pines[2,3]

[1]Department of Health Policy and Management, Milken Institute School of Public Health, The George Washington University, Washington, DC, USA

[2]US Acute Care Solutions, Canton, OH, USA

[3]Department of Emergency Medicine, School of Medicine and Health Sciences, The George Washington University, Washington, DC, USA

What Is Quality Healthcare?

What is quality in healthcare? The answer to this question is complex and varies by stakeholder, their perspective, and their connection to the healthcare system.

For patients, priorities include achieving optimal health outcomes, symptomatic relief, and ease of interacting with the system (e.g., scheduling visits and picking up prescriptions). Communication and coordination with and across clinicians (e.g., primary and specialty care) is also important, as well as having trusted relationships. For clinicians and providers, the priority is to optimize clinical outcomes. Clinicians and providers focus on ensuring care is delivered appropriately according to accepted clinical standards and available resources and that they are receiving reimbursement relative to cost and resources associated with the care provided. For health plans and payers, priorities include ensuring their enrollees achieve good health outcomes efficiently based on time and resources available through their network of clinicians and providers under a profitable business model. For state and federal regulators, priorities include ensuring large patient populations (e.g., Medicaid and Medicare) receive timely, appropriate care efficiently and within available fiscal resources. These are just four examples of the broad spectrum of stakeholders that also includes a range of state and federal healthcare agencies and programs, pharmaceutical and medical device

Quality Measurement in Healthcare, First Edition. Edited by Jesse M. Pines, Helen Burstin, and Jane Hyatt Thorpe.
© 2025 Jesse M. Pines, Helen Burstin, and Jane Hyatt Thorpe.
Published 2025 by John Wiley & Sons Ltd.

manufacturers and suppliers, ancillary providers, social services organizations, and other healthcare support networks, as well as significant variation within these groupings (e.g., from large health systems to solo physician practices), among others.

Taking these perspectives into consideration, the non-profit, independent National Academy of Medicine (NAM) defines quality as "the degree to which health services for individuals and populations increase the likelihood of desired health outcomes and are consistent with current professional knowledge [1]." The Institute of Medicine (IOM), the predecessor group for NAM, defined six key attributes of quality healthcare applicable at the individual and population levels: safety, effectiveness, patient-centeredness, timeliness, efficiency, and equity [1].

Over the last 60 years, the healthcare system has grown exponentially with expanded access to care. There have been expanded forms of insurance through the U.S. Medicare program – which primarily serves individuals aged 65 and older, as well as certain younger individuals with disabilities or specific medical conditions, as well as state-based Medicaid programs – which provide health coverage to eligible low-income individuals and families, including children, pregnant women, the elderly, and people with disabilities. Private insurance also has expanded, as have new models of care delivery and technological advances to treat and cure disease and extend longevity. This has occurred alongside the continued evolution of health and wellness as well as disease burden and a growing population that is living longer and experiencing more acute healthcare needs. In parallel, the cost of healthcare services and care delivery has increased significantly. Ongoing research consistently shows not only variation in the quality of care delivered but also disparities. There is broad variation in both access to care and quality.

In response to these trends, a quality measurement enterprise has emerged. Details of how this enterprise works are described throughout this book. Importantly, the process of how quality is measured and how quality measures are used continues to evolve. Ultimately, measurement is designed to support improvements in healthcare delivery, lead to action that results in reductions in preventable or avoidable healthcare expenditures, and improvements in equity.

What Is Healthcare Quality Measurement?

More than two decades ago, two seminal IOM reports – *To Err Is Human: Building a Safer Health System (2000)* [2] and *Crossing the Quality Chasm: A New Health System for the 21st Century (2001)* [1] – galvanized the foundation of the current quality measurement and improvement enterprise. Together they highlighted the impact of preventable errors in the American healthcare system and sparked a national call to improve the quality and decrease the rate of cost growth. Robust evidence that collectively points to the disconnect between high spending and healthcare quality and to serious deficiencies in quality has continued to fuel these efforts. The broader goal is often commonly referred to as the triple aim: (1) improving the patient experience, (2) enhancing population health, and (3) reducing per capita cost [3]. This strategy has been adopted by the U.S. Department of Health and Human Services (HHS), the Centers for Medicare & Medicaid Services (CMS), and other institutions and organizations in the private sector. More recently, an emphasis on improving the clinician experience (collectively referred to as the quadruple aim) and an emphasis on equity (collectively referred to as the quintuple aim) also have informed these goals along with patient safety and accountability.

Much work has been done to inform how to define and measure the attributes associated with quality healthcare in a meaningful way. These efforts are intended to enable consistent comparisons on metrics and to foster the development and implementation of consistent processes and structures to reduce variation and improve outcomes. This often also involves improvements for the individuals, institutions, and organizations that deliver care. Ideally, quality measurement should drive improvement in care delivery, inform clinicians and providers and consumers, and influence payment and other incentives for quality improvement. These efforts have evolved greatly over time.

Evolution of Healthcare Quality Measurement

Early Efforts

Well before the IOM work in the early 2000s, early quality measurement and improvement efforts date back to the mid-1800s, where an observant physician, Dr. Ignaz Semmelweiss, determined that handwashing prior to birthing reduced the risk of infection and mortality. Interestingly, his views were not well regarded by his peers, perhaps in part due to the caustic way he communicated [4]. Additionally, in that same period, there was a growing recognition that the spread of communicable diseases may be limited by better improving food safety and sanitation and tracking statistics. The spread of disease and the impact of poor hygiene and sanitation were increasingly clear among soldiers in tight quarters and led to efforts to improve living conditions for soldiers by Florence Nightingale and others [5].

Licensure and Accreditation (Early 1900s)

As the practice of medicine grew more organized and physicians began affiliating with hospitals, methods to monitor and regulate the delivery of healthcare also grew more sophisticated. Early licensure efforts led by physicians focused on ensuring hospitals met certain standards. One notable physician well-known for his work tracking his patients' outcomes is Dr. Ernest Codman. Codman helped organize the American College of Surgeons and the Hospital Standardization Program that ultimately became the foundation of the Joint Commission on Accreditation of Healthcare Organizations, which today assesses and accredits healthcare entities [6]. As the federal government's role in the infrastructure of delivering healthcare as well as funding for healthcare grows, so do efforts to ensure care is delivered according to set standards.

Role of Medicare/Medicaid and Federal/State Regulation (1960s/1970s)

The concept of government regulation was well established by the time the Medicare and Medicaid programs were introduced in 1965. These programs provide significant federal funding for the elderly, disabled, and low-income populations, generated in large part through tax dollars. As the Medicare and Medicaid programs grew, so did efforts to improve quality through various federally organized organizations and committees, including Utilization Review Committees (1965), Experimental Medicare Care Review Organizations (1971), Professional Standards Review Organizations (1972), Peer Review Organizations (1983), and Quality Improvement Organizations (QIO) (2002). QIOs to this day play an active role in supporting quality improvement.

The Medicare program also introduced a parallel program with standard requirements for providers, now commonly referred to as Conditions of Participation, which individual and institutional providers must meet to receive payments from Medicare. The 1970s also saw expanded application of licensure requirements to advanced practice nurses, physician assistants, optometrists, podiatrists, and psychologists. States established mechanisms to also regulate the expansion and development of new healthcare facilities through certificate of need laws designed to limit unnecessary duplication of healthcare facilities.

In 1970, the IOM – now the NAM – was established to guide health policy development and implementation based on evidence-based research across disciplines relevant to health and healthcare. The work of the IOM has played a critical role in advancing the quality efforts and initiatives over the last 50+ years. Also, during this time, a professor of methodology and governance and health services researcher, Avedis Donabedian, envisioned a more objective approach to the study of healthcare delivery and quality. His trinity of quality measurement, originally published in *The Milbank Quarterly*, described three primary methods of measuring quality that are still widely referenced today – structure, process, and outcome [7].

A structural measure is one that assesses the physical or organizational infrastructure of the healthcare system, such as resources, facilities, staff, and policies. For example, a measure may assess the number of nurses available. Process measures assess specific activities and interactions that occur in care delivery, such as diagnoses, treatments, and communication with patients. Examples may include whether a medication (like an antibiotic) was administered within a specific period of time for a serious infection. Outcome measures are the end result of healthcare delivery. Examples include whether a patient had an infection after surgery, whether a patient had functional improvement, or whether a patient lived or died following a procedure.

Growing Governmental Oversight (1980s)

The 1980s are best characterized as a period of increased governmental oversight related to quality, as concerns about quality increased in the context of new payment models. For example, the transition from a cost-based to a prospective payment system for hospitals led to concerns that Medicare beneficiaries would be discharged "sicker and quicker" because there was less of a financial incentive to keep people in the hospital for care that would not be compensated. Nursing, home health, and other long-term care providers also saw increased emphasis on quality of care with the passage of the Omnibus Budget Reconciliation Act of 1987 [8]. Early efforts to implement practice guidelines by the Agency for Healthcare Policy and Research (AHCPR) met great opposition from a sector of the physician community, as well as early efforts to report mortality rates as an indicator of quality of care by the Medicare program, National Committee for Quality Assurance (NCQA), and various states [9].

Moving Toward a National Quality Strategy (1990s)

With tensions between the role of the federal government and the role of clinicians and providers related to healthcare delivery limiting efforts, attention turned to determining what would work better in the 1990s. Work shifted away from practice guidelines to a broader focus on quality. For example, the Healthcare Effectiveness Data and Information Set (HEDIS) was launched in the 1990s by the NCQA to measure health plan performance on important dimensions of care and service [10]. Today, HEDIS measures are used by more than 90% of US health plans. Since 2008, HEDIS has also been available for use by medical providers and practices. Toward the end of the decade, the ACHPR was renamed the Agency for Healthcare Research and Quality (AHRQ), and the release of the 1998 Advisory Commission on Consumer Protection and Quality in the Healthcare Industry [11] called for a national effort to improve quality, including a recommendation for the development of a public–private partnership to foster a standardized system of quality measures. This recommendation led to the creation of the National Quality Forum in 1999 and its foundational role as a consensus-based, standard-setting organization for the review and approval of quality measures [12].

The first of the two landmark IOM reports noted above was released that same year. While most widely cited for the reference to 98,000 preventable hospital deaths a year, *To Err Is Human* emphasized that error is the result of a system of care that is organized and coordinated to prevent, recognize, and/or address problems to avoid patient harm [2]. *Crossing the Quality Chasm* issued a call for sweeping change to the healthcare system, including performance expectations, the six aims of quality improvement, and a framework to align financial incentives with quality improvements [1].

Connecting Value and Quality (2000s)

The work of the last 25 years is best characterized by ongoing efforts to incentivize quality improvement and value in the healthcare system. Numerous pieces of legislation, including the Medicare Prescription Drug, Improvement and Modernization Act of 2003 (MMA) [13], Affordable Care Act (ACA) of 2010 [14], Medicare Access and CHIP Reauthorization Act of 2015 [15], Medicare Improvements for Patients and Providers Act of 2008 (MIPPA) [16], and the Protecting Access to Medicare Act of 2014 (PAMA) [17], have authorized quality improvement programs ranging from pay for reporting programs to value-based payment models (e.g., hospital value-based payments and accountable care organizations). Quality-based payment programs now extend beyond hospitals and physicians to nursing homes, ambulatory surgery centers, and health plans and directly connect performance-based quality measurement to public reporting and financial incentives. In parallel, there also has been a proliferation of alliances and professional clinical and institutional societies that have organized to support these efforts and develop quality measures.

Since 2011, much of this work has been guided by the National Quality Strategy (NQS) authorized by the ACA and developed by AHRQ [18]. The blueprint and support for the NQS were actually developed out of the NQF's National Priorities Partnership (NPP) that brought together federal and private organizations to articulate a national vision to improve healthcare safety and people's health [19]. The NQS provides a framework that aligns priorities and levers across stakeholders.

Various motivated organizations took action to make healthcare more value-driven and banded together under the auspices of the NQF's NPP to articulate a national vision for making healthcare safer and people healthier. The dozens of federal and private entities that came together in the partnership advocated for the creation of a national blueprint for achieving a high-value healthcare system: the NQS.

The strategy embodies six priority areas and nine levers to achieve those priorities. Briefly, the **priority areas** are:

1. **Patient Safety**: Reduce harm
2. **Person- and Family-Centered Care**: Engage patient and caregivers
3. **Effective Communication and Care Coordination**: Support communication and coordination to improve patient care
4. **Prevention and Treatment of Leading Causes of Morbidity and Mortality**: Promote the most effective prevention and treatment measures
5. **Health and Well-Being of Communities**: Coordinate with communities to support health and well-being and population level
6. **Making Quality Care More Affordable**: Ensure access and affordability while reducing fraud and abuse

And the **levers** are:

1. **Measurement and Feedback**: Ensure providers and plans receive feedback on quality measurement results
2. **Reporting**: Share quality measurement results with consumers
3. **Learning and Technical Assistance**: Provide learning and training opportunities to help drive improvement
4. **Payment Models**: Reward/incentivize delivery of high-quality healthcare
5. **Certification/Accreditation/Regulation**: Ensure compliance with quality standards
6. **Consumer Incentives and Benefits**: Support informed decision-making by consumers
7. **Health Information Technology (HIT)**: Improve communication and coordination through technology
8. **Workforce Development**: Grow trained healthcare professionals aligned with quality goals
9. **Innovation and Diffusion**: Support innovative improvements across organizations

In 2022, the CMS released a similar NQS that closely aligns with AHRQ's strategy [20]. The CMS quality strategy highlights four core areas – equity and engagement, outcomes and alignments, safety and resiliency, and interoperability and scientific advancement. This strategy provides the foundation for the current quality measurement enterprise specifically for the Medicare and Medicaid programs but provides a useful reference for private sector efforts and initiatives as well.

CMS National Quality Strategy Goals

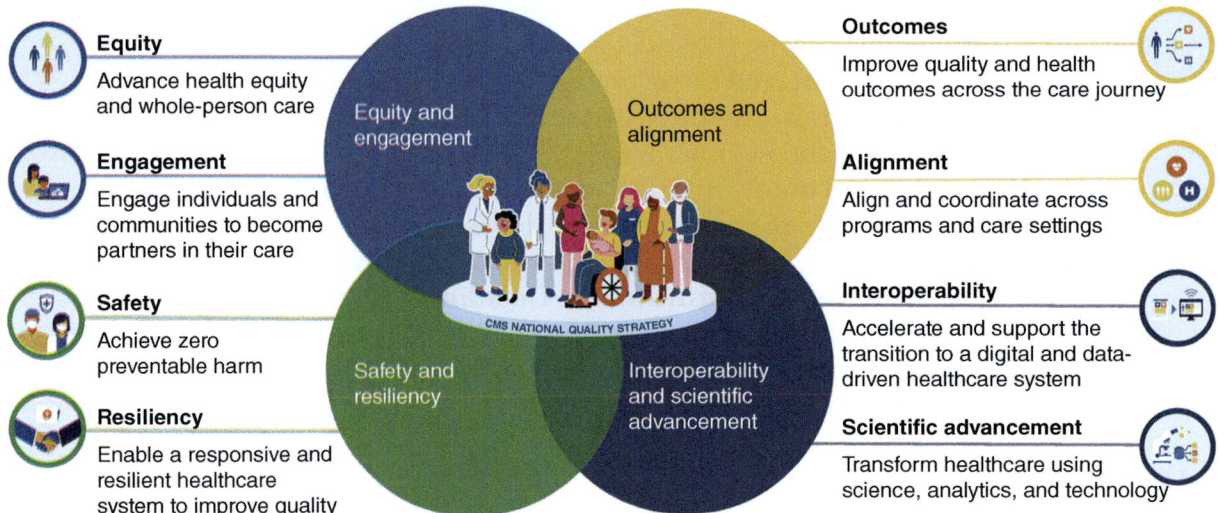

Equity

Advance health equity and whole-person care

Engagement

Engage individuals and communities to become partners in their care

Safety

Achieve zero preventable harm

Resiliency

Enable a responsive and resilient healthcare system to improve quality

Outcomes

Improve quality and health outcomes across the care journey

Alignment

Align and coordinate across programs and care settings

Interoperability

Accelerate and support the transition to a digital and data-driven healthcare system

Scientific advancement

Transform healthcare using science, analytics, and technology

Source: Centers for Medicare & Medicaid Services / https://www.cms.gov/medicare/quality/ meaningful-measures-initiative/cms-quality-strategy, last accessed on 28 January 2025 / Public Domain.

Measuring Healthcare Quality

As noted above, given the diversity of stakeholders involved in healthcare delivery, there is great variation in the definition of quality, even between and among different types of clinicians and providers (e.g., primary care physicians, specialists, and hospitals). These different priorities make what is measured and how it is measured a challenging enterprise. Appropriate, robust measurement and alignment remain elusive even with the advent of technological advances that have improved care delivery and systems of care and the capacity to collect and analyze clinical, administrative, and other forms of data to support evidence-based improvements in both. Much work to date has been focused on determining what to measure, how to measure, how to sustain the measurement effectiveness, how to utilize measurement results, and how to incentivize improvement. More recently, and importantly, considerations of equity have been introduced as a critical component of quality measurement development to identify and reduce disparities.

The chapters in this book will guide the reader through the complex elements of the quality measurement enterprise. Early chapters focus on defining a high-quality healthcare system and the use of performance data to drive quality improvement. The next set of chapters focuses on more technical elements, including how to decide what to measure, required data elements, how to develop a quality measure, how to measure cost and efficiency, measuring patient safety and patient-reported information, as well as equity. The last set of chapters focuses on integrating quality measures with payment, digital quality measurement, improving diagnostic safety, improving quality in rural settings, and workforce development. The final chapter looks ahead to the future of the quality measurement enterprise.

Discussion Questions

1.1 How do the perspectives on quality healthcare differ among patients, clinicians and providers, payers, and regulators?

1.2 Why is equity a critical component of quality healthcare measurement?

1.3 What lessons can be learned from historical advancements like handwashing and early accreditation efforts for modern healthcare quality?

1.4 How do value-based care models align financial incentives with improvements in healthcare outcomes?

1.5 What are the challenges in defining and measuring healthcare quality consistently across diverse stakeholders?

References

1 Institute of Medicine (US) (2001). *Committee on Quality of Health Care in America. Crossing the Quality Chasm: A New Health System for the 21st Century.* Washington, DC: National Academies Press (US), PMID: 25057539.

2 Institute of Medicine (US) Committee on Quality of Health Care in America (2000). *To Err Is Human: Building a Safer Health System* (ed. L.T. Kohn, J.M. Corrigan, and M.S. Donaldson). Washington, DC: National Academies Press (US), PMID: 25077248.

3 Berwick, D.M., Nolan, T.W., and Whittington, J. (2008). The triple aim: care, health, and cost. *Health Aff.* 27 (3): 759–769.

4 Zoltán, I. (2024). Ignaz semmelweis. Encyclopedia Britannica. https://www.britannica.com/biography/Ignaz-Semmelweis (accessed 18 December 2024).

5 Selanders, L. (2024). Florence nightingale. Encyclopedia Britannica. https://www.britannica.com/biography/Florence-Nightingale (accessed 18 December 2024).

6 The Joint Commission. https://www.jointcommission.org/who-we-are (accessed 18 December 2024).

7 Donabedian, A. (1966). Evaluating the quality of medical care. *Milbank Mem. Fund Q.* 44 (3) (suppl): 166–206. Reprinted in *Milbank Q.* 2005; 83(4): 691–729.

8 Public Law 100–203, Omnibus Budget Reconciliation Act of 1987.

9 National Committee for Quality Assurance. https://www.ncqa.org (accessed 18 December 2024).

10 The healthcare effectiveness data and information set. https://www.ncqa.org/hedis (accessed 18 December 2024).

11 President's advisory commission on consumer protection and quality in the healthcare industry. https://govinfo.library.unt.edu/hcquality/final/index.htm (accessed 18 December 2024).

12 National Quality Forum. https://www.qualityforum.org/about_nqf/ history (accessed 18 December 2024). See also, Burstin, H., Leatherman, S., and Goldmann, D. (2016). The evolution of healthcare quality measurement in the United States. *J. Inter. Med.* 279: 154–159.

13 Public Law 108–173, Medicare prescription drug, improvement, and modernization act of 2003. https://www.govinfo.gov/app/details/PLAW-108publ173.

14 Public Law 111–148, Patient protection and affordable care act of 2010. https:// www.govinfo.gov/app/details/PLAW-111publ148.

15 Public Law 114–10, Medicare access and CHIP reauthorization act of 2015. https://www.govinfo.gov/app/details/PLAW-114publ10.

16 Public Law 110–275, Medicare improvements for patients and providers act of 2008. https://www.govinfo.gov/app/details/PLAW-110publ275.

17 Public Law 113–93, Protecting access to Medicare act of 2014. https://www. govinfo.gov/content/pkg/PLAW-113publ93/pdf/PLAW-113publ93.pdf.

18 AHRQ National Quality Strategy. https://www.ahrq.gov/workingfor quality/about/nqs-fact-sheets/nqs-fact-sheet-0214.html (accessed 18 December 2024).

19 National Priorities Partnership. https://www.qualityforum.org/ Celebrating_the_National_Quality_Strategy.aspx (accessed 18 December 2024).

20 CMS National Quality Strategy. https://www.cms.gov/medicare/quality/ meaningful-measures-initiative/cms-quality-strategy (accessed 18 December 2024).

2 Quality Management for a High-Quality Healthcare System

Jonathan B. Perlin[1,2,3]

¹The Joint Commission/Joint Commission International, USA

²Vanderbilt University, Nashville, TN, USA

³Virginia Commonwealth University, Richmond, VA, USA

Introduction

Quality management is a fundamental aspect of healthcare delivery. Ensuring patients receive safe, effective, and timely care that meets their needs and preferences is an ethical imperative, a business necessity, and a regulatory requirement. As such, delivering high-quality care has become paramount for hospital and health system administrators and quality professionals. This chapter aims to provide a survey of the essential ingredients of a high-quality healthcare system, including the core elements of quality, mechanisms for supporting quality improvement, and the critical roles of various stakeholders and organizational governance in achieving and maintaining excellence in healthcare delivery.

Core Elements of Quality

The six aims for improved healthcare articulated in the landmark publication, "Crossing the Quality Chasm," remain a durable construct for framing and measuring performance [1]. Described in greater detail later, the aspirations include care that is:

- Safe
- Timely
- Effective

Quality Measurement in Healthcare, First Edition. Edited by Jesse M. Pines, Helen Burstin, and Jane Hyatt Thorpe.
© 2025 Jesse M. Pines, Helen Burstin, and Jane Hyatt Thorpe.
Published 2025 by John Wiley & Sons Ltd.

■ Equitable
■ Efficient
■ Patient-centered

Safety and Patient Protection

Patient safety is a foundational pillar of quality healthcare. Preventing medical errors, infections, and other adverse events that can harm patients is imperative for maintaining trust and confidence in healthcare delivery. A high-quality healthcare system implements robust safety measures, such as standardized protocols for medication administration, surgical procedures, and infection control. Establishing a culture of transparency, accountability, and continuous learning further enhances patient safety by encouraging reporting of errors, close calls, and adverse events for root cause analysis and process improvement.

While the safety of patients has been at the center of focus since the seminal publication, "To Err Is Human," the need to focus on staff and visitor safety has become increasingly critical [2]. First, patient care suffers if staff do not experience the physical and psychological safety to do their work. Second, a healing environment is simply not possible if a patient's family and other visitors fear for safety. And, finally, reports of violence in the healthcare workplace have increased multifold since before the COVID-19 pandemic [3]. Regrettably, violence includes the same issues that plague society more broadly, ranging from general incivility to threatening behavior and assaults with firearms.

Ensuring patient safety involves creating a healthcare environment where potential risks and hazards are identified and mitigated proactively. This requires a systematic approach to error prevention, including mechanisms for seeking and implementing best practices, robust reporting systems, and a culture that encourages the acknowledgment of and learning from mistakes without punitive repercussions. Patient safety protocols are designed to protect patients from preventable injuries and complications, such as infections, surgical errors, and medication mistakes.

Continuous monitoring and improvement are key components of safety in healthcare. Organizations must regularly assess their safety protocols and outcomes, adapting to new information and technologies. Training healthcare professionals in safety practices and fostering open communication among staff are essential for maintaining a safe environment. Additionally, engaging patients and their families in the safety process by educating them about potential risks and encouraging their participation in care decisions can further enhance safety outcomes, as they can act as advocates for safe practices.

Timeliness

Timeliness focuses on reducing waits and sometimes harmful delays for both those who receive and those who give care.

Timeliness in healthcare is critical to preventing conditions from worsening and ensuring optimal outcomes. Delays in treatment can lead to unnecessary physical and psychological suffering, prolonged illness, or even death. Therefore, healthcare systems must strive to reduce wait times for appointments, diagnostic tests, treatments, and procedures. This can be achieved through better scheduling practices, efficient use of resources, and the implementation of streamlined processes that minimize bottlenecks and redundancies.

Access to timely care also involves addressing logistical challenges such as transportation, appointment availability, and coordination between different levels of care. Innovations such as telemedicine and same-day appointments can help mitigate some of these challenges by providing more immediate access to care. Additionally, healthcare systems must be flexible and responsive to urgent and emergent needs, ensuring that patients receive timely interventions when they are required. Protocols for triaging acuity are necessary and must be developed and implemented in manners suited to the resources of the care environment and community need.

Effectiveness and Evidence-Based Care

Delivering care based on the best available evidence and clinical guidelines is essential for ensuring effectiveness in healthcare delivery. Evidence-based practices help healthcare providers make science-informed decisions about diagnosis and management of patient conditions, leading to improved outcomes and reduced negative variation in care. Tracking results and key performance metrics enables ongoing assessment of treatment success, aiming to improve patient results and overall care quality [1].

Effectiveness requires providing services based on scientific knowledge to those who could benefit but also refraining from providing services to those not likely to benefit. Effective care is characterized by accuracy in diagnosis, appropriate treatment plans, and the continuous evaluation of patient outcomes to ensure that interventions are achieving their intended results.

To maintain effectiveness, healthcare organizations must support ongoing education and training for their staff, promote interdisciplinary collaboration, and invest in technologies that enhance diagnostic and treatment capabilities. Moreover, effectiveness involves ongoing clinical review focused on avoiding overuse, underuse, and misuse of medical services. This means ensuring that patients receive the right care, at the right time, and for the right reasons, thereby maximizing the benefits while minimizing risks and costs.

Equity (and Access)

Ethically, access to healthcare services is a fundamental right, yet disparities in access persist across different populations. A high-quality healthcare system strives to provide accessible and equitable care to all individuals, regardless of race, ethnicity, gender and gender identity, sexual orientation, socio-economic status, geographic location, or other factors. Achieving this requires addressing barriers to access, such as financial constraints and cultural preferences, as well as providing training to the healthcare workforce.

Promoting cultural competence and sensitivity in healthcare delivery is essential to meet the diverse needs of patients from various backgrounds. This requires a commitment to understanding the social determinants of health and implementing strategies to overcome barriers that disadvantaged populations face in accessing and utilizing care. Additionally, policies and practices must be in place to ensure that resources are allocated fairly and that marginalized groups receive the support they need to achieve the same health outcomes as others. Healthcare organizations are anchor institutions in the social ecosystem. Although not resourced to solve all social vulnerabilities, they are well positioned to engage in community outreach and advocacy to address broader systemic issues that contribute to health disparities, such as poverty, education, and housing.

Efficiency and Resource Management

Efficiency in healthcare means using resources wisely to achieve the best possible outcomes without unnecessary expenditure or effort. This involves streamlining processes, reducing redundancies, and eliminating waste in all forms, including time, materials, and human resources. An efficient healthcare system maximizes the value of every dollar spent and ensures that resources are available to best meet the needs of patients, staff, and their community.

Contrary to many assumptions, quality and efficiency are not competitive interests. Meandering to the right diagnosis or therapy (when the necessary data are or could be available) is not only inefficient but a prima facie demonstration of poor performance. In the interest of both quality and efficiency, healthcare organizations must adopt evidence-based practices, leverage technology to enhance productivity, and continuously seek ways to improve workflow. This includes optimizing deployment of personnel, improving supply chain management, and using data analytics to identify areas for improvement. By focusing on efficiency, healthcare providers can reduce costs, improve patient satisfaction, and ensure that more patients can be served effectively.

Patient-Centeredness

At the heart of a high-quality healthcare system lies a commitment to patient-centered care, which places the individual and their needs at the core of the healthcare process. It emphasizes the importance of understanding each patient's unique requirements, preferences, and values and incorporating these into all aspects of care. This approach fosters a collaborative partnership between patients and healthcare providers, where patients (and, as appropriate, family members) are actively involved in their care decisions. This means that patient and family voices are heard and respected.

A patient-centered approach requires effective communication, empathy, and respect. Healthcare providers must take the time to listen to patients, provide clear and comprehensive information, and support them in making informed decisions. Additionally, patient-centered care often involves coordinating services across multiple providers and settings to support seamless and integrated care. By prioritizing the patient's experience and involving them in the care process, healthcare systems can improve patient satisfaction, adherence to treatment plans, and overall health outcomes. Moreover, data show that patients who perceive communication positively and have a more favorable experience are less likely to sue providers, even in the face of bad outcomes [4].

Mechanisms for Supporting a High-Quality Healthcare System

Quality Improvement Initiatives

Continuous quality improvement is essential for driving excellence in healthcare delivery. Quality improvement initiatives aim to proactively identify opportunities for improvement, set goals, and implement interventions to enhance the quality of care. Establishing quality improvement teams and committees engages frontline staff in quality improvement efforts, promoting a culture of continuous learning and innovation. Data analytics and performance metrics are used to track progress, identify trends, and measure outcomes, guiding decision-making and prioritization of improvement efforts.

Clinical Guidelines and Protocols

Clinical guidelines and protocols can provide evidence-based recommendations for standardizing known best care practices, thereby promoting consistency in healthcare delivery. Ideally, guidelines are developed based on the best available evidence and, where the evidence is incomplete, expert consensus. Disseminating guidelines to healthcare providers through electronic health records (EHRs), automated algorithms, clinical decision support tools, and other channels facilitates adherence to best practices. Updating guidelines regularly is necessary to ensure that care practices remain aligned with the latest evidence and recommendations.

Continuous Monitoring and Evaluation

Continuous monitoring and evaluation are essential for assessing the effectiveness of quality improvement efforts and identifying opportunities for further enhancement. Regular audits, reviews, and assessments monitor compliance with clinical guidelines, quality standards, and regulatory requirements. Collecting feedback from patients, families, and stakeholders provides valuable insights into the patient experience and helps identify areas for improvement. Benchmarking initiatives and peer comparisons allow healthcare organizations to assess their performance relative to peers and industry standards, driving continuous improvement and excellence in healthcare delivery.

Approaches to Performance Measurement and Benchmarking

Health Information Technology

Health information technology (HIT) plays an increasingly critical role in supporting quality improvement efforts and enhancing the efficiency of healthcare delivery. EHRs and other HIT systems improve documentation, communication, and coordination of care across settings. Data analytics and predictive modeling enable healthcare organizations to identify patterns, trends, and opportunities for improvement, driving evidence-based decision-making, and performance improvement. Interoperability between different HIT systems facilitates information exchange and care coordination, not only among care providers within an organization but ideally, across the environments in which patients receive care. Increasingly, patients expect access to their electronic records, and their family members are essential to assuring the integration and continuity of care requirements.

The Opportunity to Create a Learning Health System

The transition from paper to electronic records underpins the promise of a learning health system. A learning health system is a concept that emphasizes the continuous generation, analysis, and application of data to improve healthcare delivery, enhance patient outcomes, and drive innovation [5]. In a learning health system, data created through the provision of healthcare are utilized for various purposes, including improvement of quality, safety, operational management, and discovery. Predicated on the secondary use of clinical data, the opportunities a learning health system provides include:

- **Accelerating Continuous Quality Improvement**: By harnessing data from healthcare encounters, organizations can identify trends, patterns, and areas for improvement in care delivery. Analysis of clinical outcomes, patient satisfaction scores, and process metrics enables organizations to implement targeted quality improvement initiatives aimed at enhancing the effectiveness, safety, and efficiency of care.
- **Enhancing Patient Safety**: Data-driven approaches to patient safety enable organizations to identify and mitigate risks, prevent adverse events, and improve patient outcomes. Real-time monitoring of safety indicators, such as medication errors, hospital-acquired infections, and patient falls, allows for early intervention and proactive management of safety concerns, reducing harm to patients and improving overall safety culture.
- **Optimizing Operational Management**: Data analytics can inform strategic decision-making and operational management within healthcare organizations. By analyzing operational data, such as patient flow, resource utilization, and workflow efficiency, organizations can identify bottlenecks, streamline processes, and optimize resource allocation to enhance operational performance and financial sustainability.
- **Promoting Innovation and Discovery**: The rich data ecosystem within a learning health system provides opportunities for innovation and discovery. By leveraging data for research, clinical trials, and population health studies, organizations can advance scientific knowledge, develop novel treatments and interventions, and drive improvements in healthcare delivery. Collaboration between healthcare providers, researchers, and industry stakeholders facilitates knowledge exchange and fosters a culture of innovation.

In short, the utility of a learning health system is data-driven performance improvement. With the advent of machine learning (ML), patterns can be detected that can accelerate improvement in ways that are not intuitive, as ML is typically not biased by hypotheses about what does or does not work. The product of ML can be algorithms that are triggered by constellations of data, enabling the early detection of sepsis [6]. Increasingly, the promise of artificial intelligence (AI) tantalizes with the potential to dynamically offer different recommendations based on case-specific data, such as optimizing cancer therapy based on the unique features of a particular patient.

The use of data created in the process of care for research, quality improvement, or operational enhancement is referred to as the "secondary use of data." Because secondary data use is increasingly prevalent, it is essential to consider the responsible use of health data, especially in terms of disclosing data use and safeguarding patient privacy. Necessary mechanisms to appropriately disclose data use and safeguard patient interests include [7]:

- **Transparency and Informed Consent**: Healthcare organizations should clearly communicate to patients how their data will be used for quality improvement, safety monitoring, and research purposes. Patients should be provided with transparent information about data collection, storage, analysis, and sharing practices and given the opportunity to provide informed consent for the use of their data.
- **Data Governance and Security**: Robust data governance frameworks are essential for safeguarding patient data and ensuring compliance with privacy regulations, such as the Health Insurance Portability and Accountability Act (HIPAA). Organizations should implement policies, procedures, and technical safeguards to protect patient data from unauthorized access, disclosure, or misuse. This includes encryption, access controls, audit trails, and regular security assessments to identify and mitigate vulnerabilities.
- **Anonymization and De-identification**: To minimize the risk of re-identification and protect patient privacy, organizations should anonymize or de-identify patient data before use in quality improvement initiatives or research studies. This involves removing or encrypting identifiable information, such as names, date of birth, and social security numbers, while retaining essential clinical and demographic data for analysis.
- **Ethical Oversight and Institutional Review**: Research involving the use of patient data for discovery purposes should undergo ethical review and oversight by institutional review boards (IRBs) to ensure compliance with ethical principles and regulatory requirements. IRBs evaluate the risks and benefits of research studies involving patient data, assess the adequacy of consent processes, and monitor ongoing data use to protect patient welfare and privacy.
- **External Validation of Good Data Practices**: Third-party review is offered by organizations such as The Joint Commission through the "Responsible Use of Health Data" certification [8].

In summary, creating a learning health system enables healthcare organizations to harness the power of data for quality improvement, safety enhancement, operational optimization, and innovation. However, it is essential to establish mechanisms for transparent disclosure of data use to patients as well as robust safeguards to protect patient privacy and confidentiality. By promoting transparency, informed consent, and ethical data practices, healthcare organizations can build trust with patients, maintain compliance with regulatory requirements, and leverage data effectively to drive improved operating performance, as well as positive outcomes for patients and the broader healthcare community.

Roles of Stakeholders in Designing and Implementing a High-Quality Healthcare System

Interdisciplinary collaboration is key to delivering high-quality, coordinated care that meets the complex needs of patients. Because of separate reporting structures, interprofessional and interdisciplinary cultural differences, and different routes of influence, supporting dyads of physician and nursing leaders increases the effectiveness of improvement initiatives. In addition, contemporary training of pharmacists, leading to doctoral degrees, includes study of pharmacoeconomics. This translates well in linking and quantifying the desired clinical, operational, and financial outcomes. Beyond benefitting the aims of a specific initiative, interdisciplinary collaboration promotes shared decision-making, care coordination, and fosters a culture of inclusiveness, respect, and trust.

Internal Stakeholders

Healthcare Providers

Healthcare providers are at the forefront of delivering high-quality care to patients, and their engagement is essential for successful quality improvement initiatives. Ideally, clinicians deliver evidence-based, patient-centered care that meets quality standards, adhering to clinical guidelines and protocols to ensure consistency and safety in care delivery. Actively participating in quality improvement initiatives, clinicians contribute their expertise and insights to identify areas for improvement and implement evidence-based interventions that enhance the quality and effectiveness of care.

While it may seem self-evident, successful performance improvement requires physician, nursing, and other clinical leadership, as well as support from organizational administrators. Even with substantial percentages of physicians employed by their hospital or health system, physician governance still occurs under the aegis of medical staff leadership. Additionally, in contrast to nurses and other allied health professionals, as physicians progress in their careers, they do not necessarily engage in hospital or health system administrative activity. Consequently, there may be less familiarity among some physicians with an organization's quality and safety apparatus. Nevertheless, there are multiple channels for garnering physician engagement, including formal medical staff governance, hospital and departmental leadership structure, and employed physician executives (such as chief medical officers or programmatic medical directors). Importantly, some of the most compelling champions for change may be the recognized informal leaders who may have unique skill sets or wield influence through social capital in the organization.

Healthcare Administrators and Managers

Healthcare administrators and managers play a critical role in designing and implementing quality improvement initiatives that drive excellence in healthcare delivery. Setting strategic goals and priorities for quality improvement, administrators are situated to allocate resources and support for initiatives that address key areas of concern and drive improvements in clinical and operational outcomes. Monitoring performance metrics and outcomes allows administrators to assess progress and identify opportunities for enhancement, guiding decision-making and resource allocation to support continuous improvement efforts.

Patients and Families

Patients and families are vital to shaping the delivery of healthcare services and driving quality improvement efforts. As active participants in their care, patients and families can support safety and quality as advocates for their own healthcare needs and preferences, providing valuable feedback on their care experiences and suggesting areas for improvement. Engaging patients and families in shared decision-making and care planning empowers them to take an active role in managing their health and promotes patient-centered care delivery.

Including patient representatives on quality or safety committees can provide unique insights. Patients who can transcend their own care experience are especially valuable. Engaging patients and families as partners in care ensures that their perspectives and preferences are integrated into treatment plans, leading to improved outcomes and greater patient satisfaction.

Other Stakeholders

Insurers and Payers

Insurers and payers can play a significant role in shaping healthcare delivery and incentivizing quality improvement efforts. By collaborating with purchasers of care in developing performance metrics that promote accountability and align incentives with quality, providers can benefit financially from value-based contracts. Such benefits can include narrow or preferred network inclusion, premium reimbursement, and reputational value based on better measured performance in competitive markets.

More broadly, support services, such as care management and prevention programs, help improve community health outcomes, driving value for patients and payers alike. For provider organizations, such services can assist in effective patient disposition, follow up, and prevention of unnecessary readmissions.

Community Organizations and Advocacy Groups

Community organizations as well as disease and social advocacy groups can be valuable partners in promoting healthcare access, equity, and quality at the community level. Given the impact of social determinants on both health outcomes and the complexity of care provision, community organizations can be the eyes and ears of concerns that generally extend beyond the purview of formal hospital and health system responsibility.

Advocating for policies and initiatives that address social determinants of health, these organizations can work to improve healthcare access and outcomes for underserved populations and vulnerable communities by finding or funding resources, education, and support for community members. By partnering with healthcare providers, community organizations are not only stakeholders but can also drive collaboration and innovation in addressing local health needs and improving population health outcomes.

Government and Regulatory Agencies

CMS and State Health Agencies

The Centers for Medicare & Medicaid Services (CMS) and state health oversight agencies play central roles in establishing standards, regulations, and accreditation requirements that promote quality and safety in healthcare delivery. Conducting inspections, audits, and investigations helps enforce compliance and identify areas for improvement, while providing guidance, resources, and incentives supports healthcare organizations in their quality improvement efforts. As a federal agency within the US Department of Health and Human Services (HHS), CMS oversees the nation's major healthcare programs, including Medicare, Medicaid, and the Children's Health Insurance Program (CHIP). CMS's primary mission is to ensure effective, up-to-date healthcare coverage and to promote quality care for beneficiaries. Meanwhile, state health oversight agencies operate within their respective states to enforce regulations and standards that complement federal guidelines, ensuring that healthcare facilities adhere to high standards of patient care and safety.

CMS sets and enforces standards that hospitals and health systems must meet to participate in Medicare and Medicaid programs. These standards, known as Conditions of Participation (CoPs), cover various aspects of healthcare delivery, including patient rights, infection control, and the provision of care. CMS conducts regular audits and inspections, usually in collaboration with state agencies or through accreditation organizations, to ensure compliance with these standards. Hospitals failing to meet these requirements may face penalties, including the potential loss of Medicare and Medicaid funding. Additionally, CMS promotes quality through transparency initiatives such as the Hospital Compare website, which provides publicly accessible information about the quality of care in over 4,000 qualifying US hospitals. Publicly available comparative performance data tends to provide significant motivation to raise performance.

State health regulatory agencies are instrumental to enforcing state-specific health regulations and standards. These agencies, typically part of state health departments, conduct licensing and certification of healthcare facilities, ensuring they meet both federal and state requirements. They perform routine inspections, investigate complaints, and have the authority to impose sanctions on non-compliant facilities. State agencies often work in tandem with CMS to execute federal programs at the local level, ensuring a cohesive regulatory framework that upholds patient safety and care quality. Furthermore, state agencies play a crucial role in supporting emergency preparedness and response coordination with healthcare facilities to ensure readiness for public health emergencies and natural disasters. In an era of increased climate-related extreme weather threats, cyberattacks, and mass-casualty events, perpetual emergency preparedness is an essential requirement for safe healthcare operations.

Accreditation and Certification

CMS mandates that hospitals and health systems obtain accreditation from recognized accrediting organizations as a condition of participation in Medicare and Medicaid programs. This requirement ensures that healthcare providers adhere to rigorous standards of care and safety. Accreditation serves as a seal of approval that a hospital or health system meets the necessary federal health and safety standards, as outlined in the CoPs.

One of the primary accrediting organizations recognized by CMS is The Joint Commission (TJC). The Joint Commission is an independent, not-for-profit organization that accredits healthcare organizations and certifies specific clinical programs in the United States. TJC accredits a wide range of healthcare organizations, including hospitals, ambulatory care centers, nursing homes, behavioral health facilities, and home health agencies. Accreditation provides a comprehensive evaluation of healthcare facilities, focusing on key areas such as patient safety, infection control, medication management, and overall quality of care. The accreditation process involves on-site surveys conducted by experienced healthcare professionals who assess the facility's compliance with the CoPs and Joint Commission standards. These standards are developed in consultation with healthcare experts and providers, measurement experts, and patients.

Hospitals and health systems that achieve TJC accreditation demonstrate their commitment to continuous improvement and excellence in patient care. This accreditation not only helps facilities meet CMS requirements but also fosters a culture of safety and quality within the organization. Furthermore, Joint Commission accreditation is often recognized as a mark of distinction that can enhance a facility's reputation and competitiveness in the healthcare market.

In addition to accrediting healthcare organizations, the Joint Commission also certifies specific healthcare programs or services, such as stroke or behavioral healthcare. Certification signifies that a program meets rigorous standards for clinical excellence. Healthcare organizations seeking certification must demonstrate adherence to specific criteria and undergo a thorough evaluation process to ensure compliance with certification requirements.

Along with the Joint Commission, the National Committee for Quality Assurance (NCQA), Accreditation Association for Ambulatory Healthcare (AAAHC), and other organizations play vital roles in certifying healthcare organizations to ensure quality and safety standards are met. NCQA focuses on evaluating managed care organizations, health plans, and medical homes by assessing quality metrics, patient-centered care, and member experience. Through a rigorous review process, NCQA emphasizes evidence-based practices and continuous quality improvement, providing a framework for organizations to enhance care delivery. By contrast, AAAHC specializes in certifying ambulatory healthcare settings, such as outpatient surgery centers, dental practices, and community health clinics, ensuring these facilities meet standards related to patient care, safety, and operational efficiency, promoting accountability in ambulatory environments.

In summary, CMS requires hospitals and health systems to obtain accreditation from recognized organizations like the Joint Commission and others as a condition of participation in Medicare and Medicaid programs. Other types of organizations are certified by different organizations. These accreditation and certification processes ensure that healthcare providers meet rigorous standards of care and safety, ultimately promoting higher quality care for patients.

Importance of Continuous Readiness for Surveys

Continuous readiness for surveys is essential for healthcare organizations not only to achieve accreditation and programmatic certification but also as a vehicle for internally assuring constant attention to safety and quality. Several factors highlight the importance of continuous readiness:

- **Maintaining Compliance with Standards**: Healthcare organizations must adhere to established standards for patient safety, quality of care, and organizational performance to achieve accreditation and certification. Continuous readiness involves ongoing monitoring of processes, practices, and performance indicators to ensure compliance with these standards. By maintaining compliance, organizations mitigate risks, enhance patient safety, and improve overall the quality of care.

- **Identifying Areas for Improvement**: Continuous readiness enables healthcare organizations to proactively identify areas for improvement and address deficiencies before they become serious issues. Through regular self-assessments, performance monitoring, and quality improvement initiatives, organizations can identify opportunities for enhancing processes, implementing best practices, and optimizing patient outcomes. By addressing areas of weakness, organizations demonstrate their commitment to quality improvement and patient-centered care.

- **Preparing for Surveys**: Continuous readiness involves thorough preparation for surveys, including mock surveys, staff training, documentation review, and performance improvement activities. By preparing for surveys proactively, organizations can ensure a smooth survey process, minimize disruptions to operations, and maximize their chances of achieving favorable survey outcomes.

- **Cultivating a Culture of Safety and Quality**: Continuous readiness fosters a culture of safety and quality throughout the organization. By promoting accountability, transparency, and teamwork, organizations empower staff at all levels to contribute to safety and quality improvement efforts. Regular communication, education, and engagement initiatives reinforce the importance of safety and quality in daily operations and encourage staff to take ownership of their roles in delivering high-quality care.

By always maintaining compliance with standards, not just in anticipation of an impending survey, organizations can identify areas for improvement, cultivate a culture of safety and quality, and enhance their ability to deliver safe, effective, and patient-centered care.

Organizational Governance of Quality

Effective board governance is crucial for ensuring the delivery of high-quality healthcare at both the hospital and health system levels. Of course, boards of directors are instrumental in upholding the mission of an organization, constructively challenging and supporting strategic direction, and safeguarding the interests of stakeholders, including patients, staff, and the community. In the context of clinical performance, board governance encompasses several key functions essential to the assurance of quality care delivery. To be clear, as with financial propriety, this is not only a fiduciary responsibility but also a federal regulatory requirement. Because of their responsibility to the mission of an organization, boards are central to upholding the values that derive from that mission. In healthcare, that requires cultivating not only a respectful, inclusive environment but also an environment of transparency where there is both awareness of achievements and, also, attention to problems. All healthcare organizations will periodically experience adverse events. A history of transparent engagement between senior management and governance on performance issues allows organizations to work through difficult challenges constructively. More bluntly, it's better to have a transparent discussion of identified challenges than being surprised by catastrophic failure.

Boards can set a positive "tone-at-the-top" by emphasizing the importance of quality and safety in all aspects of organizational operations. Invested and informed boards can positively influence an environment where staff are empowered and expected to identify and address potential risks and opportunities for improvement. Working with leadership in aligning organizational priorities with quality improvement initiatives, boards can help ensure that resources are allocated to support initiatives aimed at enhancing the quality and safety of care.

Boards of directors are responsible for ensuring compliance with regulatory requirements, accreditation standards, and industry best practices related to quality and safety. Boards establish policies and procedures to promote compliance with quality standards and hold leadership accountable for upholding these standards. By conducting regular audits and reviews, boards can assess the organization's performance and identify areas of noncompliance, requiring corrective action as needed to mitigate risks and improve quality outcomes.

Overseeing Quality Performance

For healthcare organizations participating in federal programs such as Medicare, the governing body's fiduciary responsibility is codified under the Quality Assessment and Performance Improvement ("QAPI") regulations, which fall under the Medicare CoP [9]. The board's responsibility to oversee performance requires that boards receive regular reports on key quality indicators, clinical outcomes, patient satisfaction scores, and compliance with regulatory requirements, including:

- **Data-driven Analysis of Performance**: Hospitals must collect and analyze data on patient care, operations, and quality indicators.
- **Performance Improvement Projects**: Required projects focus on high-risk areas and must demonstrate measurable improvement.

- **Medical Error Tracking**: Hospitals must track, analyze, and implement preventive actions for medical errors and adverse patient events.
- **Executive Accountability**: Hospital leadership is responsible for ensuring the QAPI program's effectiveness and allocating necessary resources.

Of note, implementation guidance highlights that performance oversight must extend to contracted services and requires that such services meet all other CMS CoPs. While not quantified in the regulation, it is required that board oversight of quality and specific performance improvement activities must be commensurate with the complexity of the organization, reflected in board meeting minutes, and on every agenda.

By championing quality improvement initiatives, boards demonstrate their commitment to excellence in healthcare delivery and inspire confidence among stakeholders.

Effective board governance involves engaging with stakeholders, including patients, families, staff, and the community, to ensure that their perspectives and concerns are considered in decision-making processes. Boards can seek input from stakeholders through advisory committees, town hall meetings, and other fora to gain insights into the needs and expectations of the community. By fostering meaningful engagement with stakeholders, boards can better understand the unique challenges and opportunities in delivering quality healthcare and make informed decisions that align with the interests of the community.

Embracing innovation and fostering a culture of learning and adaptation can help healthcare organizations navigate change more effectively and ultimately enhance the quality of care delivered to patients. An important role for senior leadership and board governance is not only in creating an accountable environment but also in championing a learning environment that encourages organizational flexibility and openness to change in the pursuit of quality healthcare delivery.

In summary, board governance is essential to assuring quality healthcare delivery at both the hospital and health system levels. Boards set strategic priorities, establish a culture of quality and safety, oversee quality performance, support quality improvement initiatives, engage with stakeholders, and ensure compliance and accountability. By fulfilling these functions effectively, boards can contribute to the achievement of excellence in healthcare delivery and the promotion of positive outcomes for patients, staff, and the community.

Conclusion

Achieving and maintaining a high-quality healthcare system requires a multifaceted approach that addresses core elements of quality, leverages supportive mechanisms, and engages stakeholders at all levels. Mechanisms for supporting quality improvement, such as quality improvement initiatives, clinical guidelines and protocols, HIT, continuous monitoring and evaluation, and interdisciplinary collaboration, provide the infrastructure and tools necessary to drive continuous improvement and excellence in healthcare delivery. Healthcare organizations that prioritize easy-to-access and fair care, centering care around patients, ensuring safety and protection, providing effective treatments based on evidence, and managing resources efficiently are in a strong position to meet the various needs and desires of their stakeholders and patients: safe, timely, effective, equitable, efficient, and compassionate care.

Discussion Questions

2.1 How do the six aims of quality healthcare – safety, timeliness, effectiveness, equity, efficiency, and patient-centeredness – interact with each other? What are the challenges in achieving them simultaneously in a healthcare organization?

2.2 What strategies can organizations implement to foster a culture of transparency, accountability, and continuous learning to enhance patient safety? How can leadership address resistance to transparency?

2.3 The chapter highlights the importance of engaging diverse stakeholders, including patients, families, providers, and community organizations, in quality improvement initiatives. What are the benefits and challenges of involving these groups, and how can healthcare systems effectively balance their input?

2.4 The concept of a learning health system emphasizes the continuous use of data to improve care delivery. What ethical considerations should healthcare organizations keep in mind when leveraging patient data for quality improvement and research, and how can they ensure transparency and trust?

References

1 Institute of Medicine (US) (2001). *Committee on Quality of Health Care in America. Crossing the Quality Chasm: A New Health System for the 21st Century*. Washington, DC: National Academies Press (US).

2 Kohn, L.T., Corrigan, J.M., and Donaldson, M.S. (eds.) (2000). *Committee on Quality of Health Care in America, Institute of Medicine. To Err Is Human: Building a Safer Health System*. Washington, DC: National Academies Press.

3 Brigo, F., Zaboli, A., Rella, E. et al. (2022). The impact of COVID-19 pandemic on temporal trends of workplace violence against healthcare workers in the emergency department. *Health Policy* 126 (11): 1110–1116. https://doi.org/10.1016/j.healthpol.2022.09.010.

4 Stelfox, H., Gandhi, T., Orav, E., and Gustafson, M. (2005). Relation of patient satisfaction with complaints against physicians and malpractice lawsuits. *Am. J. Med.* 118: 1126–1133. https://doi.org/10.1016/j.amjmed.2005.01.060.

5 Institute of Medicine (2007). *The Learning Healthcare System: Workshop Summary.* Washington, DC: The National Academies Press.

6 Perlin, J.B., Jackson, E., Hall, C. et al. (2020). 2019 John M. Eisenberg Patient Safety and Quality Awards: SPOTting sepsis to save lives: a Nationwide computer algorithm for early detection of sepsis: innovation in patient safety and quality at the National Level (Eisenberg Award). *Jt. Comm. J. Qual. Patient Saf.* 46 (7): 381–391. https://doi.org/10.1016/j.jcjq.2020.04.006. Epub 2020 Apr 19. PMID: 32598281.

7 Accelerating Responsible Use of De-identified Data in Algorithm and Product Development. https://www.healthevolution.com/innovation-and-discovery/trust-framework-deidentified-data (accessed 12 March 2024).

8 https://www.jointcommission.org/our-priorities/responsible-use-of-health-data (accessed 12 March 2024).

9 42 CFR 482.21 QAPI regulations. https://www.ecfr.gov/current/title-42/chapter-IV/subchapter-G/part-482/subpart-C/section-482.21 (accessed 12 March 2024).

3

Clinical Quality: Deciding What to Measure

Monisha Dilip[1], Rohit B. Sangal[2], and Arjun K. Venkatesh[2]

[1]Department of Emergency Medicine, Columbia University, New York, NY, USA

[2]Yale Emergency Department, Yale School of Medicine, New Haven, CT, USA

Evidence Generation in Clinical Quality Research

The Fundamentals

Clinical research forms the bedrock of medical decision-making and provides the foundation for evidence-based medicine. This evidence is summarized in clinical practice guidelines and serves as the foundation for new quality measures or quality improvement interventions. The United States (US) Institute of Medicine – now called the National Academy of Medicine – has urged clinicians to consider six aims for quality improvement: safety, efficacy, patient-centeredness, timeliness, efficiency, and equity [1]. Ideally, clinical research would serve as the basis for any measure or intervention across these domains.

Clinical research design involves a variety of studies often selected to answer a specific research question given available resources and constraints. The study design used in the clinical research can impact the ability to answer the study question, the validity of the conclusion, and ultimately, the resulting practice guidelines and impact on patient care.

Randomized Controlled Trials

Randomized controlled trials (RCTs) are considered the gold standard in research. By randomly assigning participants to a control or experimental group, RCTs minimize selection bias and the influence of confounding factors, thereby ensuring the reliability of the results. Blinding the participant, the tester, or both to the intervention can increase the validity of the results.

If resources permit, RCTs can be conducted within a single institution or across multiple centers, sometimes across many countries. This variability allows RCTs to address a wide range of research questions, from testing the efficacy of new medications to evaluating the impact of behavioral interventions or operational changes. Despite their strengths, RCTs face limitations, including high operational costs, complex logistics, and ethical concerns over withholding potentially beneficial treatments from control groups. Given their controlled conditions, RCTs might not fully replicate real-world settings, limiting their findings' generalizability.

One prominent example of an RCT in sepsis care is the Protocolized Care for Early Septic Shock (ProCESS trial), which evaluated early goal-directed therapy (EGDT) in managing sepsis, which is the bodie's life-threatening response to infection or injury [2]. EGDT was initially introduced as a structured approach to managing sepsis, aiming to optimize blood pressure and heart rate by adjusting fluids, blood pressure medications, and oxygen delivery within the first hours of treatment. The original study by Rivers et al. in 2001 showed significant reductions in mortality with EGDT, leading to its widespread adoption and integration into sepsis guidelines [3]. However, subsequent trials such as the ProCESS trial revealed that strict adherence to EGDT did not significantly improve patient outcomes compared to standard care, demonstrating that more individualized approaches could achieve similar, if not better, patient outcomes. This dynamic nature of the medical literature over time directly informs quality measures for timely sepsis interventions and how they may change through new studies, such as early identification and antibiotic administration, which are part of implementing EGDT. This translates to patient care when clinicians and institutions focus on implementing such evidence-based practices to improve outcomes.

Historically, RCTs have been the basis for many process quality measures and quality improvement campaigns given clinician engagement with findings from strong studies.

Observational Studies

Observational studies include cohort and case-control designs. Both play a significant role in understanding the real-world effects of healthcare interventions. Cohort studies follow specific groups over time to assess the impact of various factors on health outcomes. Case-control studies compare individuals with and without a particular condition to identify potential contributing factors. Both studies are essential for investigating longitudinal outcomes and the possible contributing factors.

An example of such an observational study that informed the creation of clinical guidelines was the Peer Review Organization Voluntary Hospital Association Initiative to Decrease Events (PROVIDE) initiative, which addressed 30-day readmissions for congestive heart failure (CHF) [4]. The study evaluated interventions designed to reduce readmissions, including education and discharge planning. By retrospectively comparing hospitals that implemented the initiative with those that did not, the study identified key factors contributing to reduced readmission rates. Findings from PROVIDE were crucial in developing quality measures for CHF, specifically targeting readmission reduction strategies, which have since been incorporated into care coordination and discharge processes in hospitals.

However, the lack of randomization in observational studies can introduce potential biases since differences between the compared groups may influence the outcomes. In designing quality measures and directing quality improvement programs, such observational studies are commonly used to conduct non-experimental evaluations of an intervention (e.g., before versus after) or describe performance gaps in care processes and outcomes.

Systematic Reviews and Meta-analyses

Systematic reviews and meta-analyses summarize an existing body of literature on a specific healthcare intervention or outcome. The process begins with a clearly defined research question, followed by a systematic literature search to identify all relevant studies. This approach ensures that the data are as comprehensive as possible, increasing the reliability of the findings and minimizing the risk of bias. Meta-analyses aim to collect statistical power from multiple studies by quantitatively combining their results, making the outcomes more precise and reliable. This method is beneficial when individual studies may not provide conclusive evidence due to small sample sizes or inconsistent findings.

A prime example of how systematic reviews and meta-analyses inform guidelines is the international consensus on sepsis management, such as the Surviving Sepsis Campaign [5]. The guidelines created from this forum incorporate findings from numerous studies to formulate evidence-based recommendations for early sepsis identification and treatment. The Surviving Sepsis Campaign initially incorporated the rigid EGDT protocols as a key component of its early treatment guidelines, based on the promising outcomes from the original Rivers trial. However, as further research, including large trials like ProCESS, as described above, emerged, the campaign evolved its recommendations to emphasize more flexible, tailored approaches while still maintaining the core principles of early intervention and resuscitation. Other internationally conducted studies demonstrated that resuscitation with balanced crystalloid fluids led to a reduction in mortality in patients with sepsis [6]. These data then informed the use of early fluid resuscitation and became a cornerstone for initial sepsis bundles and the Surviving Sepsis Campaign. By synthesizing data from global studies, these guidelines focus on rating interventions like early antibiotic administration and fluid resuscitation and standardizing care across healthcare systems. This robust evidence base strengthens quality measures related to sepsis care, improving patient outcomes and reducing variability in treatment approaches.

When utilized in quality measurement, systematic reviews are often prioritized or elevated in importance because the strength of evidence is considered stronger than a single study and therefore less prone to result in quality improvement interventions with unintended consequences.

Practice Guideline Development

The Surviving Sepsis Campaign, discussed earlier, demonstrates how clinical practice guidelines are shaped by ever-changing evidence. The process of medical evidence generation, including RCTs, observational studies, and systematic reviews, forms the core of clinical practice guidelines. These guidelines synthesize the best available evidence to offer standardized recommendations for patient care. In doing so, they inform the creation of evidence-based quality measures according to the latest research, ensuring that quality improvement efforts are grounded in reliable and current scientific knowledge.

Guideline Development Process

Developing clinical guidelines is a process that requires the collaboration of multidisciplinary committees comprised of experts in a variety of fields who review the accumulated evidence, assess its quality, and formulate guidelines based on the consensus of current scientific understanding and clinical expertise. These committees can use the Grading of Recommendations, Assessment, Development, and Evaluations (GRADE) guidelines or similar local recommendations to direct their clinical practice guideline development [7]. This effort results in policies that reflect the latest research findings and consensus opinions among experts, providing clinicians with reliable and up-to-date recommendations for patient care.

Evidence Grading and Interpretation   Evidence grading enables guideline writing groups to assess the strength of a body of evidence behind a research study [8]. These grades can give clinicians, patients, and researchers valuable information about research or an assertion. Evidence can be considered high, moderate, or low strength. The Agency for Healthcare Research and Quality (AHRQ) created the Evidence-Based Practice Center (EPC), which uses the GRADE system to guide its assessments of the strength of a body of evidence [8].

The GRADE system offers a systematic approach to grading the quality of evidence and the strength of recommendations [9]. This framework evaluates evidence based on criteria such as study design, risk of bias, consistency of results, and precision. GRADE facilitates the translation of research findings into practice by providing clear, transparent, and easily interpretable guidelines for clinicians and patients. The four main aims the GRADE approach encourages are *risk of bias, consistency, directness,* and *precision.* Systematic reviewers should focus on these pillars while validating studies. The EPC, too, encourages this when assessing the strength of studies [8].

For example, in the treatment of mental health conditions during pregnancy and postpartum, evidence grading from observational studies and RCTs has informed recommendations for the use of antidepressants, considering both the benefits to the mother and potential risks to the fetus [10]. To do this, the American College of Obstetrics and Gynecology (ACOG) examined the available research studies. Because the studies performed were "RCTs with some limitations" and "observational studies without serious methodologic flaws or limitation," ACOG was able to give a strong recommendation rated with moderate-quality evidence to "initiate psychopharmacotherapy for perinatal depression or anxiety disorders." In contrast, the guidelines for the management of small intestinal bacterial overgrowth have lower-quality evidence, which results in weaker recommendations for diagnosis and certain antibiotics [11]. Like the guidelines from ACOG, the American College of Gastroenterology (ACG) has examined the evidence and found that the trials for antibiotic therapy are largely smaller clinical trials with significant flaws and heterogeneity of outcomes, resulting in lower evidence grading and therefore only a "conditional recommendation." The GRADE system allows clinicians to weigh these benefits and risks, ensuring patient-centered care in both cases.

The GRADE system's application in guideline development ensures that recommendations are based on the best available evidence, considering not only the quality of the evidence but also the balance between benefits and harms, patient values, and preferences. In quality measure development, the GRADE system is often used to establish the importance of a quality measure by serving as the evidence-based rationale regarding a specific focus of a quality measure.

Guideline Implementation and Adoption

Creating and implementing clinical practice guidelines is crucial to consistently achieving good outcomes. Implementation strategies encompass a range of activities, including increasing education for healthcare professionals, developing and disseminating digital tools and resources, and integrating guidelines into electronic health record (EHR) systems to facilitate access and adherence.

Despite best efforts, there still needs to be more consistency in how guidelines are followed across different healthcare settings. A study performed in 2003 found that only 54.9% of adults in 12 metropolitan areas received the recommended care according to clinical practice guidelines [12]. This can be due to several reasons – sometimes the guidelines need to be more relevant to specific groups of patients, there can be limited resources, or there may be some pushback against changing old habits. To tackle these issues, particular strategies are needed. This could include tailored education and training, using EHRs to remind healthcare professionals about the guidelines during patient care, or careful monitoring of how well they are being adopted and their effect on patient care.

National organizations, such as the American College of Emergency Physicians (ACEP), have created groups to recruit hospitals and specific departments to implement quality improvement initiatives and study their outcomes. The Emergency Quality Network (E-QUAL), developed by the ACEP, is an example of an initiative designed to implement clinical guidelines effectively across diverse healthcare settings [13, 14]. By offering educational resources, real-time feedback, and integration with EHRs, the network creates step-by-step guides to help emergency departments adopt best practices for conditions like sepsis, stroke, and chest pain. E-QUAL's focus on collaboration, data sharing, and continuous improvement drives more consistent adherence to evidence-based guidelines, ultimately improving patient outcomes and reducing care variability across institutions.

Effective implementation of guidelines depends on the involvement of all stakeholders in the healthcare spectrum, including policymakers, administrators, frontline clinicians, and patients. By promoting a culture of evidence-based practice and providing the necessary infrastructure and incentives for adhering to guidelines, healthcare organizations can significantly improve the quality and consistency of patient care [7].

Continuous Improvement and Adaptation

Keeping clinical practice guidelines current is critical to ensuring they stay valuable and relevant for patient care. Organizations such as the National Institute for Health and Care Excellence (NICE) in the United Kingdom (UK) set an excellent example with their structured system, which includes regularly reviewing and updating their guidelines [15]. NICE looks closely at new research and clinical data to ensure their guidelines match the latest every five years to keep abreast of changing clinical standards and new medical discoveries. This sort of continuous updating requires a robust framework for surveillance of the current evidence and deciding which topics need updating. By remaining flexible and adaptable and continuously reassessing guidelines, this process ensures that healthcare professionals make medical decisions based on the most current evidence and provide the highest quality patient care.

Analyzing the Measurable and Less Measurable Aspects of Healthcare Delivery

The effectiveness of healthcare delivery is contingent upon how well preventive services, health education, and medical care, among other factors, come together to enhance outcomes. The ability to measure these outcomes is critical for improving the quality of care and potential gaps. The following section examines the various aspects of healthcare quality measurement, including what we can and cannot quantify. However, quantifying available data, while often necessary, is insufficient to improve care quality; as Albert Einstein once said, "Not everything that can be counted counts, and not everything that counts can be counted."

The Measurable Aspects of Healthcare Delivery

Quantitative Metrics in Healthcare

The healthcare system relies on various metrics to inform policy and practice. Mortality rates are one of the most common and fundamental metrics followed globally and across healthcare settings and conditions. However, much more can be quantified, including morbidity and patient-reported outcomes. Each metric can inform the actions of organizations such as hospitals or insurance payers or change the practice of a single clinician. Quantitative metrics of quality are often characterized across the structure-process-outcome framework of Donabedian, where structural measures capture the presence of infrastructure, a fixed aspect of an institution important to high-quality care, such as hospital accreditation or the presence of an automated pharmacy dispensing unit in the hospital to reduce medication errors [16]. Process measures are more specific to a clinical action and condition and often match clinical practice guidelines, such as proportional measures of sepsis bundle compliance, which includes measures such as time to fluid and antibiotics administration and improvement of lab values such as the lactate level. Finally, outcome measures reflect a diverse set of "results" of high-quality care ranging from clinical endpoints such as mortality after an acute myocardial infarction to patient-reported outcomes such as the Seattle Angina Questionnaire after scheduled cardiac procedures to economic outcomes such as the total cost of care. Each measure type helps inform organizational and clinician quality improvement by enabling benchmarking, supporting incentives such as pay-for-performance programs, and informing public health policies [17].

Hospital readmission rates are a key indicator of the quality and continuity of care. Increasing readmission rates could highlight a potential area for improvement in discharge planning for a hospital or a review of its patient care [17]. Similarly, the length of stay in an inpatient hospital affects healthcare costs and provides insights into the efficiency of care delivery. We can also examine the cost-effectiveness of hospital care concerning medical treatments and disease management as healthcare systems strive to balance fiscal responsibility with high-quality care. Hospitals can also use patient safety indicators as a measurable outcome, such as medication error rates, hospital-acquired infection rates, and adherence to surgical checklists. These safety measures help us understand how risky a healthcare setting might be and what can be done to prevent patient harm.

Standardized Quality Metrics   Quality measures can be standardized in measurement and reporting to facilitate benchmarking and other comparative endeavors. In the realm of healthcare payers that are often compared and even reimbursed based on quality measures, the Healthcare Effectiveness Data and Information Set (HEDIS), developed by the National Committee for Quality Assurance, has long provided the foundation for common measurements based on administrative insurance claims data sources [18]. Similarly, patient experiences of hospital care are captured using standardized surveys such as the Hospital Consumer Assessment of Healthcare Providers and Systems (HCAHPS) [19]. These surveys allow us to examine patient experience in various interactions, including communication with doctors and nurses, hospital staff responsiveness, and cleanliness. These surveys are standardized to allow for large amounts of data aggregation and comparison across different healthcare providers and systems. By quantifying these aspects, we can create a foundation for evaluating and improving healthcare delivery. Hospitals and policymakers can leverage quantitative metrics to identify areas of strength and opportunities for improvement to target interventions that can enhance quality of care, improve patient safety, and boost cost-effectiveness.

While nearly 1,000 such quantitative quality measures have been evaluated for national use over the past 20 years, much of healthcare still needs to be measured by national quality measurement and payment programs. Furthermore, there is an increasing federal emphasis on parsimony in quality measurement to favor focused improvement on high-priority areas. These include maternal health, patient safety, and healthcare disparities, which have reduced the number and breadth of quality measurement and improvement programs in hospitals and other healthcare facilities.

The Less Measurable Aspects of Healthcare Delivery

In contrast to the measurable aspects of healthcare delivery, the qualitative features can present a more nuanced view. These factors include personal experiences, ethical concerns, and cultural issues, which contribute to the quality of care delivered but cannot be easily quantified in a reliable and valid way.

Qualitative Dimensions of Healthcare

Patient Experience   Patient experiences can be highly subjective and encompass a variety of perceptions based on the care they receive – from emotional support to how well their providers communicate. Not only can these factors affect patient satisfaction, but they can also impact outcomes [20]. For example, an association was discovered between hospital mean patient satisfaction scores and surgical outcomes, including a significantly reduced relative risk and lower odds of death for the hospitals with the highest mean patient satisfaction scores. Measuring provider communication or the subjective aspects of patient experience is difficult. While HCAHPS may assess aspects of these critical outcomes, most healthcare system interactions do not consider or track a patient's experience across a journey of illness or care. Future quality measurement efforts are likely to move beyond surveys and utilize novel analyses of qualitative reviews, as online resources such as Yelp often capture and present such data to patients and caregivers seeking to evaluate healthcare providers. Initial online surveys such as "Rate My Doctor" or even ratings on Google allow patients to review their clinicians and hospitals subjectively, laying the foundation for future similar resources.

Cultural Competency   Cultural competency refers to the ability of providers to effectively deliver care that meets patients' social, cultural, and linguistic needs [21]. This becomes especially important for minority groups because cultural differences can result in discrepancies in understanding that can change the quality of care. It is challenging to measure the cultural competency of an individual provider or a healthcare system and its impact on a patient population; however, emerging tools that utilize technologies such as ambient listening offer the opportunity for routine clinical interactions to be measured across known as well as newly developed measures of patient comprehension, and cultural sensitivity, among other aspects.

Ethical Considerations   Ethical considerations like patient autonomy and upholding informed consent are fundamental to high-quality care and patient rights. However, measuring these ethical practices is more complex since they involve complex and nuanced judgments. Recently, the Centers for Medicare & Medicaid Services (CMS) unveiled a structural measure of the informed consent process. The transition toward digital consent tools may permit future measurement opportunities embedded within clinical delivery.

Systemic and Environmental Factors

Healthcare Equity   Healthcare equity involves assessing access to care and equal quality of care across different patient populations, especially underserved groups. Because there are many factors to consider, including socioeconomic status, geographic location, and racial/ethnic identities, all of which can affect access to care to different degrees, selecting targets for health equity improvement can be daunting. In healthcare quality measurement, an increasing number of quality measures and quality improvement (QI) interventions are reporting quality scores or results stratified by race or ethnicity to ensure that disparities are not masked and that efforts directed at care improvement help all subgroups of patients. For example, studies have shown that African American women experience higher rates of preeclampsia and worse outcomes compared to other groups [22]. Quality metrics that track blood pressure monitoring and timely intervention can reveal disparities in maternal outcomes between racial and ethnic groups. Healthcare organizations can target interventions such as early screening and education programs to reduce these disparities and improve health equity across populations.

Interdisciplinary Collaboration and Teamwork   Interdisciplinary collaboration among healthcare professionals, between various specialties in the hospitals, and between different types of staff is critical to maintaining quality of care [23]. Communication forms the basis of many errors. However, assessing the quality and impact of this cooperation poses a challenge. Researchers try to use a variety of proxies to simulate communication, such as markers for teamwork and role clarity. For example, a collaborative approach to reducing central line-associated bloodstream infections (CLABSI) involves clear communication among physicians, nurses, and infection control teams to ensure adherence to insertion and maintenance protocols. By examining where communication breakdowns occurred and implementing teamwork-based strategies, hospitals have significantly lowered CLABSI rates [24]. Still, standardization becomes problematic, given the variety of interactions and personality types.

Evaluating Quality Measures

Implementing quality measures allows us to evaluate the effectiveness of different healthcare improvement interventions. Ultimately, the goal is to utilize quality measures to align practice with a healthcare organization's overarching mission and broader objectives for healthcare delivery.

Understanding Quality Measures

Quality measures allow us to benchmark and assess clinical outcomes, patient safety protocols, and patient experience to assess the quality of healthcare delivery. Selecting quality measures for quality improvement should be grounded in the existing evidence base and understanding of the desired setting for intervention as well as a logic model capable of linking a given quality measure to practice change or care actions that will yield the desired improvement. To meet this goal, a quality measure must be scientifically sound and relevant to the care setting and clinicians measured.

Decision-Making Framework

Selecting the most appropriate quality measures requires a structured approach. This decision-making framework is critical for healthcare providers aiming to implement quality measures effectively. It encompasses several vital stages:

1. **Assessment of Current Performance**: The first step involves assessing the system's current state. This assessment identifies performance gaps and areas where patient care could be improved. By understanding the current state of healthcare delivery, organizations can pinpoint specific domains that require attention.

2. **Goal Setting**: After identifying areas for improvement, the next step is to set clear, achievable goals (such as SMART goals). SMART goals are **S**pecific, **M**easurable, **A**chievable, **R**ealistic, and **T**ime bound. These objectives should be directly linked to the areas identified in the initial assessment phase.

3. **Selection of Quality Measures**: The next step is to identify and implement quality measures that align with the previously noted goals. The selected measures should provide insights into progress toward the set goals, enabling healthcare providers to monitor advancements and adjust strategies as necessary.

This decision-making framework emphasizes a systematic approach to creating and selecting quality metrics. By systematically assessing the current state of care, setting targeted objectives for improvement, and carefully selecting measures that align with these goals, healthcare providers can ensure that their efforts are focused and effective. This framework also lays the groundwork for continuous improvement goals, offering a mechanism to track progress toward achieving high care quality standards.

External bodies, such as CMS and the Joint Commission, also play a role in setting quality metrics for US hospitals. These organizations establish standardized measures that healthcare providers must meet to ensure compliance with national standards. For instance, CMS tracks metrics like 30-day readmission rates for conditions like heart failure, as discussed earlier [25]. Similarly, the Joint Commission measures adherence to surgical safety protocols. These external benchmarks help hospitals associate their internal quality improvement efforts with broader regulatory requirements and industry best practices.

Healthcare organizations can foster a culture of quality improvement through this structured approach. The selection and implementation of these quality measures is a very meticulous process. The framework above ensures that chosen metrics support organizational goals, meet patient needs, and adhere to regulatory standards.

Considerations for Selecting Quality Measures

Alignment with Organizational Goals

Quality measures should match the organization's mission and strategic goals. This alignment ensures that improvement efforts directly contribute to the organization's stated aims, such as improved outcomes, enhanced patient care, or improved operational efficiency. Increased alignment can also mean a more concerted effort to mobilize resources and focus resources on where they can have the most impact.

Patient-Centered Care

Patient-centered care and satisfaction remain the mainstay of most healthcare organizations. Therefore, patient care should be considered when evaluating quality measures to use within the organization. This consideration underscores the importance of including measures that assess patient experiences, outcomes, and the quality of communication and interaction with healthcare providers.

Data Availability and Integrity

Data availability and integrity can make implementing a quality measure difficult or straightforward. Most healthcare systems have robust data collection and analysis systems that can be used to track performance in quality metrics. These systems ensure that the measures chosen can be reliably tracked over time, providing a valid basis for assessing performance and identifying areas for improvement.

Regulatory and Accreditation Requirements

Healthcare organizations must operate within a regulatory framework and often have specific quality measures already dictated for compliance. Ideally, these measures are aligned with recognized standards and best practices. Accrediting bodies such as the Joint Commission may set additional benchmarks, so internal quality measures must at least reflect these.

Cost-Effectiveness

Creating these systems to track and implement the previously mentioned quality measures is likely costly. Thus, measures should be evaluated for cost-effectiveness, and preferences should be given to those that provide economic benefits upon implementation with low burden and management costs.

Challenges and Solutions in Implementing Quality Measures

Challenges

Implementing the quality measures can pose some challenges that can impede progress and potential effectiveness, thereby lessening the impact. Some setbacks can include limited resources, including financial, technological, and personnel, during the implementation and monitoring of the quality measures. In addition, resistance to change within the organization can impede improvement initiatives, as members are reluctant to change long-standing practices or adopt new protocols. After implementation, managing, storing, and analyzing the data can pose a challenge to the organization, making it difficult to gain actionable insights.

Potential Solutions

To overcome these challenges, healthcare organizations can employ some solutions:

- **Engaging Stakeholders**: Actively engaging all relevant stakeholders, including staff and clinicians, in new quality measures can help foster a culture of quality improvement. Doing so ensures buy-in and facilitates identifying and resolving barriers to implementing quality measures.
- **Leveraging Technology**: As discussed above, using advanced technological solutions, such as EHRs, data analytics platforms, and patient management systems, especially in conjunction with one another, can significantly enhance data management difficulties. This can improve accuracy and efficiency, resulting in more effective tracking of quality measures.
- **Adopting Best Practices for Change Management**: As discussed above, resistance to change can hinder the adoption of quality measures. Implementing best practices in change management can address this resistance to change. This involves clear communication about the benefits of quality measures and demonstrating the positive impact of changes on patient care and the organization itself.

Conclusion

Choosing and implementing quality measures are key steps toward achieving high-quality healthcare. Through this chapter, we have emphasized adopting a systematic and evidence-based approach to quality measurement that considers quantitative and qualitative data to understand how healthcare is being delivered and where there is room for improvement. As the current healthcare landscape continues to evolve, so must the methods we use to measure and improve the quality of care.

New technologies, such as data analytics, artificial intelligence, and machine learning, are opening new frontiers in healthcare. They help refine the accuracy of quality measures and widen the scope of outcomes, allowing for a deeper understanding of how effective the care delivered is and the patient experience. It is essential for healthcare organizations and their clinicians to continue their commitment to innovation and to be adaptable to new approaches for quality improvement. By embracing new technologies, healthcare providers can ensure that their services meet and exceed care standards, improving outcomes.

Discussion Questions

3.1 The chapter highlights the importance of using evidence from RCTs, observational studies, and systematic reviews to develop quality measures. How can healthcare organizations ensure they effectively translate these research findings into practice, especially in rapidly evolving fields like sepsis care?

3.2 RCTs are often seen as the gold standard for clinical research but come with limitations like cost and logistical complexity. What are alternative methods for evidence generation to support quality measurement and improvement, and how can their findings be validated for real-world application?

3.3 Despite the availability of clinical practice guidelines, adoption of evidence-based care remains inconsistent across healthcare settings. What barriers prevent the implementation of evidence-based guidelines, and how can quality measurement help?

3.4 The chapter mentions the difficulty of quantifying aspects like patient experience and cultural competency. How can healthcare systems incorporate both measurable and qualitative factors into their quality improvement efforts to provide holistic care?

3.5 With advancements in technology such as artificial intelligence and machine learning, what ethical considerations should be addressed to ensure that these tools are used responsibly in healthcare quality measurement and improvement?

References

1 Institute of Medicine (US). Committee on Quality of Health Care in America (2001). *Crossing the Quality Chasm: A New Health System for the 21st Century*. Washington, DC: National Academies Press, 337 p.

2   Pro, C.I., Yealy, D.M., Kellum, J.A. et al. (2014). A randomized trial of protocol-based care for early septic shock. *N. Engl. J. Med.* 370 (18): 1683–1693.

3   Rivers, E., Nguyen, B., Havstad, S. et al. (2001). Early goal-directed therapy in the treatment of severe sepsis and septic shock. *N. Engl. J. Med.* 345 (19): 1368–1377.

4   Graff, L., Orledge, J., Radford, M.J. et al. (1999). Correlation of the Agency for Health Care Policy and Research congestive heart failure admission guideline with mortality: peer review organization voluntary hospital association initiative to decrease events (PROVIDE) for congestive heart failure. *Ann. Emerg. Med.* 34 (4 Pt 1): 429–437.

5   Evans, L., Rhodes, A., Alhazzani, W. et al. (2021). Surviving sepsis campaign: international guidelines for management of sepsis and septic shock 2021. *Intensive Care Med.* 47 (11): 1181–1247.

6   Rochwerg, B., Alhazzani, W., Sindi, A. et al. (2014). Fluid resuscitation in sepsis: a systematic review and network meta-analysis. *Ann. Intern. Med.* 161 (5): 347–355.

7   Khodambashi, S. and Nytro, O. (2017). Reviewing clinical guideline development tools: features and characteristics. *BMC Med. Inform. Decis. Mak.* 17 (1): 132.

8   Singh, S., Chang, S.M., Matchar, D.B. et al. (2012). Chapter 7: grading a body of evidence on diagnostic tests. *J. Gen. Intern. Med.* 27 Suppl 1 (Suppl 1): S47–S55.

9   Busse, R., Klazinga, N., Panteli, D. et al. (eds.) (2019). *Improving Healthcare Quality in Europe: Characteristics, Effectiveness and Implementation of Different Strategies.* Copenhagen, Denmark: European Observatory on Health Systems and Policies.

10 (2023). Treatment and management of mental health conditions during pregnancy and postpartum: ACOG clinical practice guideline No. 5. *Obstet. Gynecol.* 141 (6): 1262–1288.

11 Pimentel, M., Saad, R.J., Long, M.D. et al. (2020). ACG clinical guideline: small intestinal bacterial overgrowth. *Am. J. Gastroenterol.* 115 (2): 165–178.

12 McGlynn, E.A., Asch, S.M., Adams, J. et al. (2003). The quality of health care delivered to adults in the United States. *N. Engl. J. Med.* 348 (26): 2635–2645.

13 Venkatesh, A.K., Scofi, J.E., Rothenberg, C. et al. (2021). Choosing wisely in emergency medicine: early results and insights from the ACEP emergency quality network (E-QUAL). *Am. J. Emerg. Med.* 39: 102–108.

14 Zachrison, K.S., Ganti, L., Sharma, D. et al. (2022). A survey of stroke-related capabilities among a sample of US community emergency departments. *J. Am. Coll. Emerg. Physicians Open* 3 (4): e12762.

15 Duffield, S. and Jonsson, P. (2023). The real-world impact of National Institute for Health and Care Excellence's real-world evidence framework. *J. Comp. Eff. Res.* 12 (11): e230135.

16 Donabedian, A. (2005). Evaluating the quality of medical care. 1966. *Milbank Q.* 83 (4): 691–729.

17 Atkinson, J.G. (2020). Improving quality measurement: design principles for quality measures. *J. Ambul. Care Manage.* 43 (2): 100–105.

18 Mainous, A.G. 3rd and Talbert, J. (1998). Assessing quality of care via HEDIS 3.0. Is there a better way? *Arch. Fam. Med.* 7 (5): 410–413.

19 Ellenbogen, M.I., Ellenbogen, P.M., Rim, N. et al. (2022). Characterizing the relationship between hospital google star ratings, hospital consumer assessment

of healthcare providers and systems (HCAHPS) scores, and quality. *J. Patient Exp.* 9: 23743735221092604.

20 Sacks, G.D., Lawson, E.H., Dawes, A.J. et al. (2015). Relationship between hospital performance on a patient satisfaction survey and surgical quality. *JAMA Surg.* 150 (9): 858–864.

21 Truong, M., Paradies, Y., and Priest, N. (2014). Interventions to improve cultural competency in healthcare: a systematic review of reviews. *BMC Health Serv. Res.* 14: 99.

22 Force, U.S.P.S.T., Bibbins-Domingo, K., Grossman, D.C. et al. (2017). Screening for preeclampsia: US preventive services task force recommendation statement. *JAMA* 317 (16): 1661–1667.

23 Wei, H., Horns, P., Sears, S.F. et al. (2022). A systematic meta-review of systematic reviews about interprofessional collaboration: facilitators, barriers, and outcomes. *J. Interprof. Care* **36** (5): 735–749.

24 Pate, K., Brelewski, K., Rutledge, S.R. et al. (2022). CLABSI rounding team: a collaborative approach to prevention. *J. Nurs. Care Qual.* 37 (3): 275–281.

25 Faillace, R.T., Yost, G.W., Chugh, Y. et al. (2018). Is 30-day mortality after admission for heart failure an appropriate metric for quality? *Am. J. Med.* 131 (2): 201. e9–201.e15.

II How Do We Measure Quality in Healthcare?

4

A Primer on Quality Measurement Development

Heidi Bossley

Bossley Consulting, LLC, Alexandria, VA, USA

Measure Development

The Basics of Quality Measures

Measure Types

Quality measure development starts with an idea or concept, and that concept traditionally follows the framework developed by Donabedian [1] with the measure focused on a structure, process, or outcome.

Structure measures are "the relatively stable characteristics of the providers of care, of the tools and resources they have at their disposal, and of the physical and organizational setting in which they work" [1]. These types of measures determine whether the necessary infrastructures are in place such as participation in a registry or whether a facility has established the needed components to satisfy a specific topic (e.g., equity, patient safety). Unlike the other two measure types, structure measures are not reported at the patient level; rather, they are captured through a yes/no attestation across the clinician, facility, or other group on which you are evaluating quality (measurement entity).

Process measures examine "a set of activities that go on within and between practitioners and patients" [1]. They will determine whether an assessment, medication, or procedure is provided to a specified set of patients such as aspirin at arrival to a hospital when suffering from a heart attack.

Outcome measures assess "changes in a patient's current and future health status that can be attributed to antecedent health care" [1]. Readmissions or mortality are two traditional examples of outcome measures. Outcomes may also be more intermediate and examine markers of health status such as achievement of a specific blood pressure level for patients with a diagnosis of hypertension.

When we think of quality measurement, we typically view these metrics as ones that measure clinical aspects of care such as the delivery of a

Quality Measurement in Healthcare, First Edition. Edited by Jesse M. Pines, Helen Burstin, and Jane Hyatt Thorpe.

treatment or medication or the achievement of a specific clinical outcome. There is an increasing degree of interest and development of measures that provide information on the quality of care from a patient's viewpoint. These measures are labeled as patient-reported outcome performance measures (PRO-PMs) and are derived from the "report of the status of a patient's health condition that comes directly from the patient, without interpretation of the patient's response by a clinician or anyone else" [2]. PRO-PMs still fit within the Donabedian framework of structure, process, and outcome and center on whether your goal is to establish a process of collecting PRO data (structure), determine how many patients within a practice completed the PRO survey in a given timeframe (process), or evaluate the degree to which that practice was able to achieve either a specific threshold score or some other clinically significant finding (outcome).

Intended Use

Regardless of the focus of the measure, it is important to determine its intended use – quality improvement only versus accountability. Measures used for quality improvement purposes are intended for internal use. For example, a hospital sees an increase in their infection rates and a root cause analysis shows that clinicians are not performing specific processes that could contribute to a reduction in those rates. In this instance, the hospital will be using the results of the measure to create educational tools and internal improvements and does not plan on publicly reporting the results or comparing performance against other facilities. As a result, they may be less concerned about the level of evidence supporting the concept and will not worry if the results are not reliable and/or valid. On the other hand, if the measure will be used to assess performance and promote accountability of an entity through public reporting, accreditation, or some incentive-based payment, the stakes become higher and there is diminished tolerance for a measure that falls short of meeting a minimum set of criteria: the measure must be firmly anchored in evidence, precisely specified for its data source, feasible and reliable to ensure that results can be repeated across the measurement entities, validly reflect evidence-based care, and the results are transparent.

Understanding your goal (quality improvement only vs. accountability) is critical from the start since developing measures for accountability requires greater rigor, detail, and resources. The rest of this chapter assumes that accountability is the intended use.

Building Blocks of Quality Measures

Before we get to the details on measure development steps, we should first discuss the building blocks of quality measures. The components of a measure (i.e., numerator, denominator, exclusions/exceptions, timeframes, attribution) must be well-defined (Table 4.1).

Table 4.1: Measure components and examples.

Measure component	Example [3]
Measure description ■ Statement describing the patient population and the aspect of care to be measured in a given timeframe ■ It is in essence a high-level summary of the population of interest (denominator) and measure focus (numerator)	Percentage of patients aged 18 years and older with a diagnosis of heart failure (HF) with a current or prior left ventricular ejection fraction (LVEF) ≤40% who were prescribed or already taking ACE inhibitor or ARB or ARNI therapy during the measurement period
Denominator ■ Defines the population of interest supported by the evidence during a specified time period ■ May be focused on patients with a specific diagnosis or on procedures that are performed	All patients aged 18 years and older with two qualifying encounters during the measurement period and a diagnosis of heart failure with a current or prior LVEF ≤40%
Numerator ■ Aspect of care – structure, process, or outcome – being measured and its frequency	Patients who were prescribed or already taking ACE inhibitor or ARB or ARNI therapy during the measurement period
Exclusions ■ Those patients for whom the aspect of care does not apply ■ Exclusions are considered absolutes where the aspect of care is consistently not appropriate for a set of patients ■ These patients are removed from the denominator even before you look to see if the numerator is met	Patients with a history of heart transplant or with a left ventricular assist device (LVAD) prior to the end of the outpatient encounter with moderate or severe LVSD

Exceptions
■ Those patients for whom the aspect of care does not apply
■ Exceptions are not absolute and are intended to be used at the provider's discretion based on patient characteristics or choice
  ■ We look to see if the numerator is met first
  ■ If not, then we look to see if an exception is documented
  ■ If one is, then we remove the patient from the denominator
	Documentation of medical reason(s) for not prescribing ACE inhibitor or ARB or ARNI therapy (e.g., pregnancy, renal failure due to ACEI, allergy, intolerance, other medical reasons)
	
	Documentation of patient reason(s) for not prescribing ACE inhibitor or ARB or ARNI therapy (e.g., patient declined, other patient reasons)

Denominator timeframe ■ Period of time in which the patient population will be captured	**Denominator timeframe** ■ During the measurement period (e.g., within a 12-month period)
Numerator timeframe ■ Period of time in which the clinical action occurs	**Numerator timeframe** ■ Ordered or currently taken during the same measurement period
Attribution ■ Determination of how a patient or set of patients is assigned to the measurement entity (e.g., clinician, facility)	Patients have two qualifying encounters during the measurement period Rationale: The requirement of two or more visits is used to establish that the eligible professional or eligible clinician has an existing relationship with the patient.

$$\frac{Numerator}{Denominator - Exclusions + Exceptions}$$

Figure 4.1: The formula used to calculate performance scores.

Performance scores are then calculated (Figure 4.1).

Performance scores may also be risk-adjusted or risk-stratified (e.g., sorting and displaying the scores by well-defined categories or characteristics), particularly if the focus is on a patient outcome. Risk models or stratification should be based on evidence and validity, and these approaches are intended to account for underlying patient risk (e.g., pre-existing conditions, social determinants of health) for which the measure entity cannot likely control or influence [4].

In addition, it is important to determine the "who" – the level of measurement (e.g., individual clinician, facility, community/region), and the "where" – the settings of care (e.g., acute care facility, ambulatory/outpatient clinics, home health), and both of which should be closely linked to the intent of the measure.

By defining all of these components from the start and refining throughout the development process, you will be able to create precise specifications that outline the data elements and associated coding and carefully select the appropriate data source and testing of the data.

All of these building blocks serve critical roles in ensuring that the measure as specified is feasible to collect and will produce reliable and valid results.

Measure Development Lifecycle

Measure development and maintenance is a continuous process or lifecycle (Figure 4.2). In this section, the fundamental steps are discussed, but the order and timing of the various stages may differ depending on what resources and funding are available and at what points during the process. Measure developers also continue to identify new tools and collaboratives such as test beds that enable them to iteratively define and specify the measures based on real-time feedback and expert panel input including patients and caregivers. While it remains unclear whether cost savings could be realized through some of these initiatives, the benefits may be more likely to be seen during implementation where the measure is demonstrated to be feasible, reliable, and valid from the beginning.

Several helpful resources are available during the development process. Centers for Medicare and Medicaid Services (CMS) offers the Measures Management Hub (https://mmshub.cms.gov/) with information on the Blueprint Measure Lifecycle and related tools. CMS also provides templates and access to the CMS Measures Inventory Tool (https://cmit.cms.gov/cmit/#/) to identify similar measures when focused on aligning quality measures with their programs. The Partnership for Quality Measurement (https://p4qm.org/)

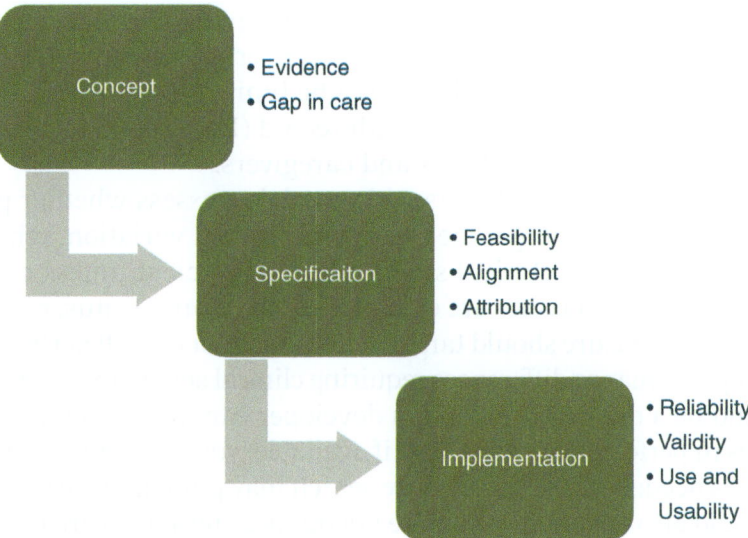

Figure 4.2: Measure development lifecycle.

serves as the consensus-based entity (CBE) for measure endorsement and offers guidance and criteria on endorsement in addition to the annual review of potential measures for consideration for use by CMS, which is now called the pre-rulemaking measure review (PRMR).

Concept Development

Measure development starts with a focus on a specific disease or condition or desire to improve a specific process or outcome. At this point in the process, narratives of the measure components outlined in Table 2.1 are created and refined based on clinical input.

Measure concepts should be defined based on clinical evidence. The evidence supporting this concept could be from a clinical practice guideline, systematic reviews, or other sources. Specifically, if an outcome is the focus, then there should be at least one structure or process that is demonstrated to be able to drive improvements in that outcome and any process of interest should be proximal to the outcome, which will increase the likelihood that the measure can encourage improvement. If the measure is a PRO-PM, then it should target a symptom or other variable deemed most meaningful by patients. Consistency in conclusions from cited literature and guidelines is essential, and any measure intended for CBE endorsement and/or CMS quality programs should align with the criteria and expectations of these groups.

Refining the concept to ensure that it is aligned with the evidence can be accomplished through multiple avenues including convening a set of experts such as a Technical Expert Panel (TEP), conducting focus groups, surveys, or other methods to vet the clinical concept, and through validity testing.

The degree to which this vetting process is formalized is not as critical as ensuring that the right people with the right expertise are consulted throughout the process. These experts should not be limited to clinicians and could include groups such as electronic health record (EHR) vendors if electronic data will be leveraged and patients and caregivers.

In the initial development phase, it's crucial to assess whether potential gaps in care exist. Creating a measure with limited variation, where most providers already meet clinical standards, is inefficient unless disparities among patient characteristics are evident (e.g., insurance status, race/ethnicity). Ideally, the measure should target areas with poor overall performance or significant performance differences requiring clinical action. In a perfect world, there would be a data set on which a developer can query and determine if differences in performance exist, and if available, you can begin to evaluate if a measure is needed. If not, a literature search may pinpoint true gaps in care.

You should also ensure that you are not duplicating a measure that already exists or is similar to your concept. The CMS Measure Inventory Tool (CMIT), the CMS Quality Payment Program (QPP) Qualified Clinical Data Registry (QCDR) measure file, and the Partnership for Quality Measurement (PQM) Submission Tool and Repository (STAR) are good resources to begin to identify whether a similar measure exists.

Measure Specification Development

Once you have defined the measure components and drafted your narratives based on the evidence reviews and clinical input, specifications are then created. Measure specifications must be aligned with the "who" and "where" and include clear narrative statements, definitions, and logic to define data elements or data collection as needed, relevant coding (e.g., ICD-10-CM, CPT®, LOINC®, SNOMED CT, RxNorm), and risk models. All of this information ensures that the measure is well-defined and precisely specified. This level of detail contributes to a measure that is reliable – one that can be consistently implemented across providers and sites and valid – the specifications reflect the underlying evidence and measure intent.

The relevant coding is from data sources that are available to the entity to which the measure is attributed and in the appropriate care settings. Data sources can include administrative data (e.g., claims), EHR data, other digital data sources such as laboratory or pharmacy, patient-generated health data, paper medical records, and surveys such as PROs.

At this point in the process, data feasibility assessments should begin. The aim is to evaluate the collection feasibility and potential burden of data used for denominator, numerator, and other measure components. This iterative process involves testing sites, input from clinical experts at the point of care, or other methods to determine data source viability and extraction efforts across providers and sites. User feedback during this phase may prompt adjustments to specifications. Harmonizing data element definitions and codes across measures is encouraged to alleviate the data collection burden for end users.

In instances where the data source is EHRs or other digital data, it is important to determine the extent to which each data element is in structure fields (availability), the degree to which the data element is extracted from the original source (accuracy), whether there are associated codes (e.g., ICD-10-CM, CPT) available, and if the collection of each data element requires changes in clinical workflows and data capture – is the "juice worth the squeeze" (workflow). This information should be captured for each data element across multiple EHR vendor systems using the electronic clinical quality measure (eCQM) feasibility scorecard [5].

Several tools and resources are available that can assist with measure specification and coding development, all of which can be accessed through the Electronic Clinical Quality Improvement (eCQI) Resource Center [6], including:

- Measure Authoring Development Integrated Environment (MADiE) [7]
    - This new environment replaces the Measure Authoring Tool (MAT) and Bonnie tools, which allows the development and testing of eCQMs using that allows using the newest data standards.
- Value Set Authority Center (VSAC) [8]
    - The central repository of value sets (i.e., code sets) is maintained by the National Library of Medicine. In addition to allowing users to create and maintain value sets, it can also serve as a great resource to adopt existing value sets for use.

As reliance on digital data for measure development grows, understanding how to leverage data standards is crucial. Health Level 7 (HL7) International, a standard development organization for healthcare data, plays a key role. HL7 oversees various activities, with two pertinent data standards being Clinical Quality Language (CQL) [9] for harmonizing eCQMs and clinical decision support and FHIR [10] for open-source standards in data exchange. The transition is expected for all eCQMs and eventually digital quality measures (dQMs) to adopt the FHIR standard. Additionally, alignment with the US Data for Interoperability (USCDI) [11], a set of standardized data elements for health information exchange overseen by the Assistant Secretary for Technology Policy/Office of the National Coordinator for Health Information Technology (ASTP/ONC), can be expected over the next few years.

Measure Implementation

After defining narratives and specifications, the next step involves assessing the scientific acceptability of a measure before full implementation. This evaluation determines whether the draft measure will yield reliable and valid performance scores. Reliability, characterized by the repeatability or precision of measurement [12], is assessed to determine how well a measure can be applied across providers and sites based on specifications. Validity, indicating the correctness of measurement [12], assesses how accurately the measure captures its intended target. Scientific acceptability is evaluated at both the individual data element level and across performance scores, with varying purposes, processes, and resource requirements at each testing level (refer to Tables 4.2 and 4.3).

The measure's intended use, attribution, data source, and other attributes all contribute to these determinations, and while reliability and validity address distinct questions, they are also intertwined (Figure 4.3). Developers and end users often face tradeoffs and decisions. For instance, if a required data element is less valid due to capturing it being burdensome, developers must decide whether to revise the measure or if the effort is justified. Similarly, if the scores are less reliable due to small sample sizes but the measure shows potential to drive improvement, a decision is needed regarding moving forward with implementation. Ideally, a measure that is intended to be used for accountability would achieve a high level of reliability and validity.

After evaluating the testing results and modifying the measure specifications, it is time for the measure to be rolled out and implemented. During this shift, funding and other resources are often reduced, but a developer's work is never done. The evaluation of the measure and its continued relevance and accuracy should be ongoing, and developers must ensure that its intent

Table 4.2: Reliability testing.

Level	Data element	Measure score
Purpose	Evaluates whether data elements are consistently collected across providers and sites	Determines how precise the performance scores are
Process	Typically accomplished through inter-rater reliability where the same specifications are provided to two data abstractors and rates of agreement across the two are compared	Typically accomplished through signal-to-noise analyses where performance scores are analyzed for the amount of error
Data and resources required	Precise specifications, trained data abstractors, and testing partners willing to provide access to patient medical records	Data (counts of numerators, denominators, and exclusions/exceptions) are aggregated at the measurement entity level across multiple groups
	Requires statistician to complete the analysis	Requires statistician to complete the analysis

Table 4.3: Validity testing.

Level	Data element	Measure score
Purpose	Assesses the degree to which the individual data elements are correct	Assesses the degree to which the measure correctly reflects the quality of care provided
Process	Typically compares the agreement of the individual data elements against another authoritative source For example, eCQM testing requires a comparison of an electronic report of the measure results against the gold standard (patient medical record) across several vendor systems	Typically accomplished through: 1. Face validity and/or 2. Empirical validity Face validity requires a formal survey of relevant clinical experts assessing their agreement that the measure as specified reflects clinical evidence and can be used to distinguish differences in quality Several options to test the empirical validity of a measure are available including correlations to other quality measures that are conceptually related (e.g., decreased hospital readmissions are correlated with cost reductions)
Data and resources required	Testing partners provide de-identified patient-level data as well as access to the authoritative source Requires data abstractors and a statistician to complete the analysis	Face validity: set of experts to complete the survey and results are summarized Empirical validity example: aggregated scores for the measure of interest as well as the aggregated data for at least one other correlated measure Requires statistician to complete the analysis

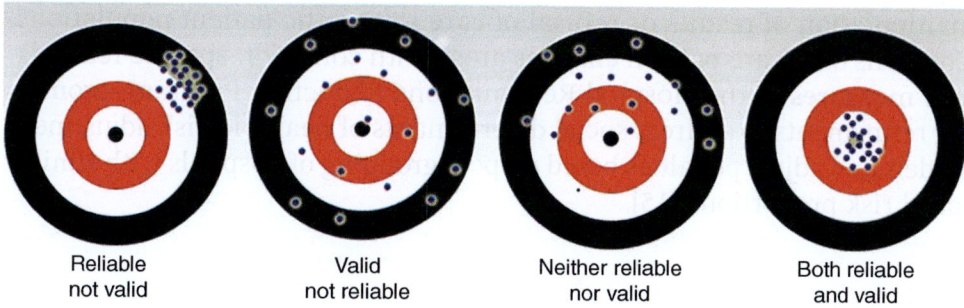

| Reliable
not valid | Valid
not reliable | Neither reliable
nor valid | Both reliable
and valid |

Figure 4.3: Inter-related concepts of reliability and validity.

continues to be aligned with clinical evidence and the coding and other specifications remain up to date. Coding updates are usually completed annually with a full maintenance review (e.g., evidence review, retesting) occurring periodically (e.g., three years).

Developers and end users should evaluate its potential for true quality improvement (frequently referred to as the use and usability of a measure). These evaluations of year-over-year performance scores are more easily accomplished for measures that are in programs where benchmarking or public reporting occurs (e.g., clinical registry, CMS quality program). Feedback from end users on how they are able to leverage the measure to drive improvements at the point of care and/or opportunities to refine the specifications can be invaluable.

Developers are also asked to determine whether the measure once implemented produced any unintended consequences. Regrettably, the absence of any negative reports on a measure often leads groups to conclude that the measure is working as intended, which may or may not be true. It is the responsibility of any developer to actively monitor whether the measure could be encouraging or incentivizing changes in practice patterns that could negatively impact patient care and/or outcomes.

Unintended negative consequences based on a measure's design (e.g., misaligned with evidence or poorly specified) or implementation (e.g., its use in a program incentivizes care stinting) can arise, and measures should not knowingly encourage treatment leading to misuse, underuse, or overuse of services. One such example is a measure on whether patients with community-acquired pneumonia were prescribed antibiotics within the first four hours of admission. During the initial implementation by CMS and The Joint Commission, experts voiced concerns with the limited evidence that was used to set the four-hour time window and the potential unintended consequences of a clinician rushing to diagnosis to meet the time requirement as well as possible antibiotic overuse [13, 14]. This measure was modified to attempt to address the issues but eventually was removed from the programs due to these concerns. Other well-designed measures can produce negative results, especially in pay-for-performance programs, incentivizing manipulation of results or refusal of care to specific patient populations. Concerns over care pattern changes arose with condition-specific readmission measures in the Hospital Readmissions Reduction Program, prompting refinements to address social determinants of health in risk adjustment models and adjust penalties based on peer grouping of hospitals with similar social risk proportions [15].

Discussion Questions

4.1 How do you think Donabedian's framework influences the way quality measures are developed? Can you think of real-world examples where each type of measure is most effective?

4.2 What are some potential challenges and benefits of integrating PRO-PMs into clinical quality improvement programs?

4.3 The chapter highlights the importance of determining whether a measure is for quality improvement or accountability. How might the intended use of a measure influence its design, implementation, and evaluation processes?

4.4 The chapter describes examples of unintended negative consequences, such as antibiotic overuse due to rigid time requirements in pneumonia treatment measures. How can developers anticipate and mitigate potential unintended consequences when designing quality measures?

4.5 The reliability and validity of a measure are critical for its success. What trade-offs might developers face when balancing reliability, validity, and feasibility during the measure development process? How would you prioritize these factors in a new measure for a high-stakes accountability program?

References

1 Donabedian, A. (1980). *The Definition of Quality and Approaches to Its Assessment*. University of Michigan.

2 Guidance for Industry Patient-Reported Outcome Measures: Use in Medical Product Development to Support Labeling Claims (2009). https://www.fda.gov/media/77832/download.

3 Heart Failure (HF): Angiotensin-Converting Enzyme (ACE) Inhibitor or Angiotensin Receptor Blocker (ARB) or Angiotensin Receptor-Neprilysin Inhibitor (ARNI) Therapy for Left Ventricular Systolic Dysfunction (LVSD) 11.1.000. ecqi. healthit.gov.https://ecqi.healthit.gov/sites/default/files/ecqm/measures/CMS135v11.html (accessed 24 September 2024).

4 Hanna, C. *Issue Brief Health Risk Assessment and Risk Adjustment in the Context of Health Equity Key Points*. https://www.actuary.org/sites/default/files/2022–08/RiskAdjust.8.22.pdf (accessed 23 November 2023).

5 P4qm.org (2023). https://p4qm.org/sites/default/files/2023–08/eCQM–Feasibility–Scorecard.xlsx (accessed 24 September 2024).

6 eCQI Resource Center (2022). https://ecqi.healthit.gov/.

7 MADiE. https://madie.cms.gov (accessed 24 September 2024).

8 Value Set Authority Center. https://vsac.nlm.nih.gov/ (accessed 24 September 2024).

9 Clinical Quality Language (CQL). https://cql.hl7.org/ (accessed 24 September 2024).

10 Index – FHIR v4.0.1. https://www.hl7.org/fhir/index.html.

11 United States Core Data for Interoperability (USCDI) | Interoperability Standards Advisory (ISA). https://www.healthit.gov/isa/united–states–core–data–interoperability–uscdi.

12 National Quality Forum. Guidance for Measure Testing and Evaluating Scientific Acceptability of Measure Properties (2011). https://www.qualityforum.org/WorkArea/linkit.aspx?LinkIdentifier=id&ItemID=70943 (accessed 24 September 2024).

13 Baum, S.G. and Kaltsas, A. (2008). Guideline tyranny: primum non nocere. *Clin. Infect. Dis.* 46 (12): 1879–1880. https://doi.org/10.1086/588302.

14 Wachter, R.M., Flanders, S.A., Fee, C., and Pronovost, P.J. (2008). Public reporting of antibiotic timing in patients with pneumonia: lessons from a flawed performance measure. *Ann. Intern. Med.* 149 (1): 29–32. https://doi.org/10.7326/0003-4819-149-1-200807010-00007.

15 Chapter 1: Mandated report: The effects of the Hospital Readmissions Reduction Program (June 2018 report) (revised November 27, 2019). MedPAC. https://www.medpac.gov/document/http-www-medpac-gov-docs-default-source-reports-jun18_ch1_medpacreport_rev_nov2019_v2_note_sec-pdf/ (accessed 24 September 2024).

5 Data Requirements for Valid Quality Measurement

Jeffrey Geppert, Brenna Rabel, and Ian Warmbrodt

Battelle, Columbus, OH, USA

Introduction

Data are the backbone of quality measurement. Without accurate, complete, and timely data, it is impossible to reliably and validly assess healthcare quality. Data used in quality measurement come from a variety of sources, each contributing unique insights into different aspects of care delivery [1].

The purpose of this chapter is to explore the critical role of data in the development and implementation of valid quality measures, with a particular focus on the evolving demands of digital measurement. As healthcare continues to advance toward a more data-driven and technology-enabled environment, understanding data requirements for quality measurement is more important than ever. This chapter delves into the foundational aspects of quality measurement, examines the specific data quality requirements necessary for valid measurement, and discusses the unique challenges and opportunities associated with digital quality measurement.

Foundations of Quality Measurement

Goals of Quality Measurement

Clinical quality measurement (CQM) aims to evaluate and enhance the effectiveness, safety, and patient-centeredness of healthcare. Ideally, this process would encompass the entire care continuum, from prevention to outcomes, assessing adherence to evidence-based standards and best practices. The goal is to achieve optimal health outcomes, better value, improved quality of life, fewer disparities, and reduced harm.

Quality Measurement in Healthcare, First Edition. Edited by Jesse M. Pines, Helen Burstin, and Jane Hyatt Thorpe.
© 2025 Jesse M. Pines, Helen Burstin, and Jane Hyatt Thorpe.
Published 2025 by John Wiley & Sons Ltd.

In an ideal scenario, unfettered by data limitations, CQMs would capture nuanced patient outcomes like whether a patient recovered as expected after an acute illness like pneumonia, functional status after a debilitating condition like stroke, symptom relief from an acute painful condition like a fracture, and health equity which assesses whether people from different races and socioeconomic status receive similar care and treatments. Other key aspects would include care coordination as people transition across settings, the quality of communication between the patients and clinicians, the degree of patient engagement in their care, and longitudinal outcomes like one-year or even five-year mortality after treatment. Social determinants of health, such as housing stability and food security, which can contribute to health outcomes, would also be considered, alongside care value metrics like cost, efficiency, and waste reduction. Real-time data would facilitate continuous learning, rapid cycle improvement, and personalized medicine, enabling healthcare systems to optimize care delivery, policy, and research for better health, care, and value [2].

History and Limitations of Quality Measure Data

The ability to achieve the goals of quality measurement is limited by the types of data and extraction methods available. Besides the necessity of data that are accurate, complete, and timely, optimal quality measurement also requires interoperable electronic health record (EHR) systems where EHRs share data with one another so that patients can be tracked throughout their care journey, from outpatient clinics, inpatient settings, and post-acute care settings. Without this, it is difficult, if not impossible, to reliably evaluate longitudinal outcomes or even certain types of care coordination as patients transition across settings of care.

The history of CQMs reflects both the evolution of health information technology (Health IT) and the ongoing tension between benefits and burden (Figure 5.1). Historically, CQMs were based mainly on two data sources: administrative (billing or claims) data and manual patient chart abstraction. The advantage of administrative data was that these data were universally available, inexpensive to use, and structured based on national standards (e.g., International Classification of Diseases [ICD-10-PCS] [3]). Administrative claims data only assesses patient demographics, diagnoses, and billed treatments. While comprehensive and accessible across settings, a disadvantage of quality measurement is that the data are not collected to track clinical outcomes. As such, there is a marked absence of clinical specificity that would be needed to meaningfully assess clinical quality. In contrast, manual chart abstraction from clinical notes in the medical record had essentially the reverse set of advantages and disadvantages. These data were clinically detailed, but selectively available, expensive to collect due to the necessary reliance on manual abstractors,

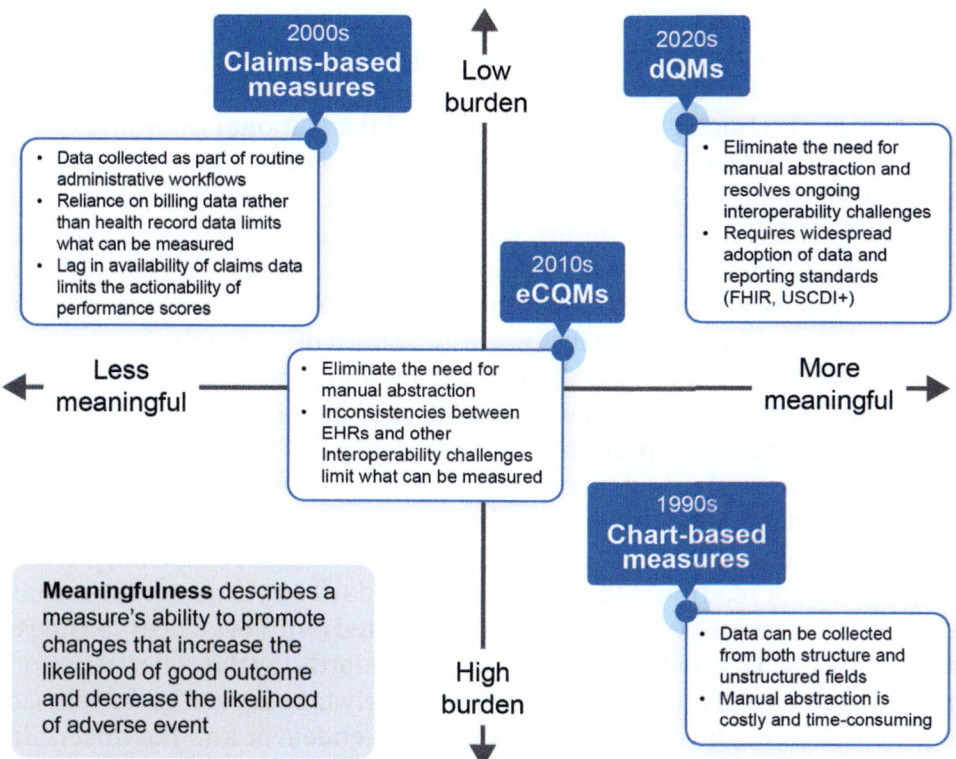

Figure 5.1: Historically, healthcare quality measures have been derived from manually abstracted medical record data, administrative claims, or digitally extracted medical record data, all of which are associated with important burden–benefit trade-offs.

and largely unstructured (being derived from notes or non-standardized structured fields).

With the advent of EHR data and other Health IT solutions came the rise of electronic CQMs (eCQMs), a type of quality measure reliant on electronically extracted structured medical record data [4]. These measures were intended to retain the advantages and mitigate the disadvantages of administrative data and manual patient chart abstraction. This was based on the assumption that widespread adoption of EHRs would lead to the availability of accurate, standardized, and electronically extractable data for use in quality measurement. The experience to date, however, has been mixed. Universal data availability across settings is limited by the absence of routine and systematic interoperable and complete health information exchange (HIE). EHR data capture remains primarily focused on documenting and directing clinical care delivery and justifying billing. Any addition to support quality measurement is often poorly integrated into the clinical workflow and adds to the expense. The adoption of national clinical standard terminologies for the purpose of measurement is sometimes constrained by the absence of a compelling business case to do so.

Digital quality measures (dQMs)[1] represent the next phase of quality measurement [5]. To address the barriers impeding eCQMs, both the Centers for Medicare & Medicaid Services (CMS) and the recently named Assistant Secretary for Technology Policy and Office of the National Coordinator for Health IT (ASTP/ONC) have promoted the adoption and implementation of two modern standards in Health IT known as the US Core Data for Interoperability (USCDI) for data capture [6] and the Health Level Seven International's (HL7®) Fast Healthcare Interoperability Resources (FHIR®)[2] for data exchange [7]. By addressing both workflow (USCDI) and interoperability (FHIR), these standards have the potential to both decrease the burden and increase the benefit of quality data collection and reporting. However, the trade-off of standards is that the quality "space" defined by these standards will reflect the clinical "space" that is measurable and therefore improvable. The burden of standard adoption (the costs of implementing the standard in EHR systems, for example) should be justified in terms of the benefit of improved quality of care and outcomes for patients (lower mortality, fewer complications or readmissions). Generally, standard implementers are reluctant to allocate resources without a well-supported (with evidence) "business case." Both USCDI and FHIR are evolving standards for the collection, storing, and exchange of data elements that will likely take several more years to be widely adopted, given the complexity of the endeavor and the uncertain benefit–burden trade-off.

Standards for terminology, interoperability, and logic are necessary building blocks for a bottom-up approach to CQM development. However, consensus-based approaches – making choices based on the use cases identified by interested parties compared to an engineering approach with an explicit benefit–burden calculation – to the development of these standards have resulted in unintended consequences such as increased data entry and extraction costs, interruptions in clinical provider workflows that disrupt care pathways and detract from time with patients, and the failure to address gaps in care through timely feedback to providers and patients. Efforts to align and harmonize the technical and structural approach to CQMs are intended to decrease these burdens and to integrate the technical workload into existing systems. However, there is nothing built into these processes to ensure that the resulting measures are reliable, valid, feasible, and useful. So, the historical tensions between benefit and burden will continue and will be informed by recent work on quantifying the burden of documentation in healthcare [8].

---

[1]CMS defines digital quality measures (dQMs) as quality measures that use standardized, digital data from one or more sources of health information that are captured and exchanged via interoperable systems; apply quality measure specifications that are standard-based and use code packages; and are computable in an integrated environment without additional effort (https://ecqi.healthit.gov/dqm).

[2]FHIR is a standard for healthcare data exchange, published by HL7® (https://www.hl7.org/fhir/).

Universal Data Requirements

All quality measures, regardless of their data collection methodology, rely on data that are accurate, complete, timely, and consistent. The section below describes these universal data requirements in greater detail.

Accuracy and Precision

Accuracy is the cornerstone of any quality measurement system. In the context of healthcare, accuracy refers to the degree to which data correctly reflect the real-world situations or events it is intended to capture. Precise data, on the other hand, consistently reproduces the same values across multiple measurements under unchanged conditions. Together, accuracy and precision ensure that the data used in quality measurement are reliable and trustworthy.

Inaccurate or imprecise data can lead to incorrect conclusions about the quality of care, potentially resulting in misguided decisions that could negatively impact patient outcomes and healthcare delivery. For instance, errors in data entry, coding inaccuracies, or incorrect patient information can distort the results of quality measures, making it appear that a provider is performing better or worse than they are. To mitigate these risks, healthcare organizations must implement rigorous data validation processes, such as regular audits, cross-checks with external data sources, and the use of standardized coding practices.

Completeness

Completeness refers to the extent to which all required data elements are present and accounted for in a dataset. Incomplete data can lead to significant gaps in quality measurement, making it difficult to draw accurate and meaningful conclusions. For example, if a quality measure relies on data from EHRs, but key information such as lab results or medication histories is missing, the measure may not accurately reflect the quality of care provided.

Ensuring data completeness is particularly challenging in healthcare, where information is often spread across multiple systems and sources. Patients may receive care from different providers who use different EHR systems, leading to fragmented data that are difficult to aggregate and analyze. To address this challenge, healthcare organizations must prioritize data integration and interoperability, ensuring that data from various sources can be combined to create a complete and accurate picture of patient care.

Timeliness

Timeliness refers to the availability of data when it is needed for decision-making. In healthcare quality measurement, timely data are essential for identifying and addressing issues as they arise, rather than after the fact. However, many existing quality measures rely on delayed or outdated data which can severely restrict the ability to respond promptly to quality concerns, potentially jeopardizing patient safety and care outcomes. For instance, if data on patient outcomes are only available months after care has been delivered, it becomes difficult to intervene effectively and prevent adverse events for future patients.

To improve timeliness, healthcare organizations must focus on enhancing real-time data collection and reporting systems, leveraging digital tools such as EHRs and HIEs to capture and share data as soon as it is generated. While progress has been made, the gap between data generation and availability continues to hinder proactive quality management and continuous improvement efforts.

Consistency

Consistency refers to the uniformity of data across different sources, systems, and time periods. Inconsistent data can lead to unreliable quality measures, as variations in data collection methods, definitions, or coding practices can result in discrepancies that obscure the true quality of care. For instance, if two different hospitals use different criteria to define a hospital-acquired infection where a patient develops an infection in the hospital, comparing their infection rates would not provide a valid assessment of quality.

Achieving consistency requires the standardization of data collection and reporting practices across the healthcare system. This includes adopting common definitions and coding standards, such as those provided by the ICD, a standard naming system for diseases, or the Logical Observation Identifiers Names and Codes (LOINC) system, a standard naming system for laboratory tests. Additionally, training and education for healthcare professionals on data entry and management are essential to ensure that data are consistently recorded and interpreted.

Requirements for Electronically Reported Data

To achieve the requirements detailed above, electronically reported measures have additional requirements to make up for the lack of a manual abstractor to clean and interpret the data, including structured data fields that are coded using standard terminologies, and assertions that those structured fields are routinely and consistently used to store relevant data.

eCQM and dQM Standards

eCQM standards are crucial to the successful electronic capture of measure data. Within the context of Health IT, standards are the agreed-upon methods and terminology for defining healthcare data elements and enabling data reporting. From a data quality perspective, the most relevant standards are those related to data element definitions and interoperability.

Standards to Define Data Elements

To enable electronic data capture, all data elements necessary to calculate a measure score must be coded using a nationally recognized terminology standard, such as Systematized Nomenclature of Medicine – Clinical Terms (SNOMED CT), which is the global language for clinical terms, or RxNorm [9], which is a standardized naming system for drugs. A value set is a list of terms and their associated codes, used to describe clinical and administrative concepts. Value sets provide groupings of unique values along with a standard definition from one or more standardized vocabularies used to describe the same concept. The National Library of Medicine maintains the Value Set Authority Center (VSAC) [10], which serves as the official source of value sets for eCQMs used in CMS programs.

The USCDI is an evolving standard for the collection and storing of data elements, but it is not yet widely adopted. However, its primary use will be in conjunction with FHIR to enable the capture of dQMs. The overall process for defining a standard from information collected during routine care is depicted in Figure 5.2.

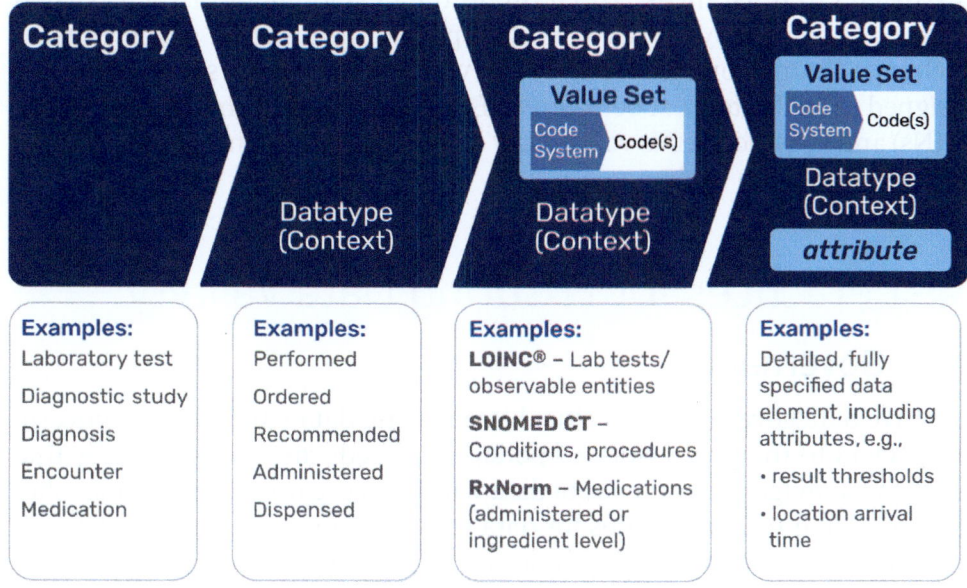

LOINC® – Logical Observation Identifiers Names and Codes

Figure 5.2: To define a standard, categories of information are cross-walked against generic data types, which are then defined using code sets. These code sets are further specified with attributes to become executable standards. Source: QDM - Quality Data Model / Electronic Clinical Quality Improvement Resource Center, https://ecqi.healthit.gov/qdm?qt-tabs_qdm=about, last accessed on 28 January 2025 / Public Domain.

Interoperability Standards

As mentioned above, CMS and ASTP/ONC have jointly promoted the adoption of USCDI (for data capture) and FHIR (for data exchange). These standards enable dQM data capture and reporting beyond what is possible with eCQMs.

FHIR provides a standard-based application programming interface (API) that enables authorized users to access, exchange, and use health information. FHIR provides a set of industry-curated data elements through web-based FHIR "resources," which group together different data that have a common theme (e.g., healthcare service). FHIR by itself does not ensure a standard for collecting and storing data elements. Therefore, HL7 has published a US Core Implementation Guide (IG) that instructs health IT systems on how to map common data elements to FHIR, including those from USCDI.

Trusted Exchange

Besides data collection (USCDI) and exchange (FHIR), the third requirement for electronically reported data is privacy and security. The Health Insurance Portability and Accountability Act (HIPAA) of 1996, Public Law 104-191 [11], included provisions requiring national standards for electronic healthcare transactions and code sets, unique health identifiers, and security. In general, these standards may limit the interoperability of healthcare data outside of trusted circumstances. To facilitate the development of such trusted circumstances, the ASTP/ONC has supported the creation of the Trusted Exchange Framework [12]. The Framework is a common set of principles designed to facilitate trust between HIEs and Health Information Networks (HINs) and by which HINs voluntarily elect to comply to enable efficient and secure information exchange.

Best Practices for Ensuring Data Validity

Data Governance

Effective data governance is critical to ensuring data validity. Data governance refers to the framework of policies, procedures, and standards that guide the management and use of data within an organization. It establishes clear roles and responsibilities for data stewardship, ensuring that data are collected, stored, and used in a manner that preserves their accuracy and integrity. Effective data governance is a collaborative effort that requires input and cooperation across various levels of an organization, including:

- **Chief Information Officer (CIO)**: Often oversees data governance efforts and makes sure they align with the organization's strategic goals.

- **Chief Data Officer (CDO)**: In some organizations, this role specifically focuses on managing data and setting rules for how it should be used.
- **Data Governance Committee**: A cross-functional team made up of staff from various departments (e.g., clinical, IT, compliance, and operations) that creates and enforces rules for data management.
- **Data Stewards**: Staff members who take care of the data they handle, making sure it's accurate and follows established rules.
- **Compliance Officers**: Ensure that the organization's data practices follow laws and regulations.
- **IT Department**: Provides the technology and systems needed to manage and protect data.

A strong data governance framework begins with the establishment of clear data standards and definitions. Consistency in how data elements are defined and recorded across different systems and departments is essential for maintaining data validity. For example, standardized coding practices, such as the use of ICD-10 codes for diagnoses or LOINC codes for lab results, help ensure that data are interpreted consistently, regardless of where or by whom it is recorded.

Data governance also involves the creation of data quality monitoring processes. Regular audits and data quality checks can identify errors or inconsistencies in the data, allowing organizations to address issues before they impact quality measurement. Additionally, data governance should include protocols for data access and security, ensuring that only authorized personnel can access sensitive data, which help prevent unauthorized changes or breaches that could compromise data validity.

A good example of data governance is the ASTP/ONC HIT Module Certification program [13], which allows software developers to certify their health IT modules by demonstrating their adherence to a set of functional requirements. Receiving this certification signals that the health IT module – for example, a patient portal – possesses the baseline capabilities required to enable electronic data collection and reporting.

Data Validation

Data validation is the process of verifying that data are accurate, complete, and consistent before they are used in quality measurement. Several techniques can be employed to validate data, each addressing different aspects of data quality.

One common data validation technique is cross-validation, where a measure developer compares data from one source with data from another source to ensure consistency. For example, patient demographic data recorded in an EHR can be cross-validated with data from a HIE to ensure accuracy. Discrepancies between the two sources can indicate errors that need to be addressed, either in the data element definitions in the measure specification or in the EHR workflows for how information is documented (which might be suggested in the measure's implementation guidance). Often data validation involves comparing one data element to a "gold-standard" data element that has been previously validated. Such studies use metrics such as sensitivity, specificity, positive predictive value (PPV), and negative predictive value (NPN) to quantify the degree of "validity."

Another effective technique is the use of automated data validation tools. These tools can flag potential errors in real time, such as missing data elements or outlier values that fall outside expected ranges. Automated validation tools are particularly useful in large datasets where manual validation would be impractical. By identifying and correcting errors as they occur, these tools help maintain data validity throughout the data collection process.

In addition to automated tools, manual data validation methods, such as peer reviews or audits, can also play a vital role in ensuring data validity. For example, a peer review of clinical documentation can identify inconsistencies or inaccuracies in how data are recorded, which can then be corrected before the data are used in quality measurement.

Training and Competency

Ensuring data validity is not solely the responsibility of data governance structures and validation tools. It also requires a well-trained and competent workforce. Healthcare professionals who are responsible for data entry, management, and analysis must understand the importance of data validity and be equipped with the skills necessary to maintain it.

Training programs should focus on educating staff about data standards, coding practices, and the specific requirements of the quality measures they are working with. Regular training updates are essential to keep pace with changes in technology, regulations, and best practices. For example, as new versions of EHR systems are implemented, staff should be trained on any changes to data entry processes or validation procedures that could affect data validity.

Competency assessments can also help ensure that healthcare professionals are adequately prepared to handle data management tasks. These assessments can include practical exercises that test the ability to accurately enter and validate data, as well as knowledge tests on relevant data standards and best practices. By ensuring that staff are competent in these areas, healthcare organizations can significantly reduce the risk of data validity issues.

Case Studies and Examples

Illustrating the practical application of the principles and best practices discussed in previous sections, this chapter includes two case studies. These examples provide valuable insights into how data quality, governance, and validation play out in real-world scenarios.

Case Study 1: Traditional Quality Measurement in Infection Control

The first case study examines a hospital's effort to improve infection control through traditional quality measurement methods. The hospital, a mid-sized urban facility, was experiencing higher-than-average rates of surgical site infections (SSIs). In response, the hospital leadership implemented a quality improvement initiative aimed at reducing SSIs by adhering to evidence-based guidelines.

Data Collection and Measurement. The hospital relied on a combination of manual chart reviews and administrative data to measure compliance with SSI prevention protocols. Key data elements included the timely administration of prophylactic antibiotics, adherence to sterile techniques, and proper postoperative wound care. These data were collected by a team of infection control nurses who manually reviewed patient records and entered the relevant information into a centralized database.

Challenges and Solutions. One of the primary challenges the hospital faced was ensuring the accuracy and completeness of the data collected. Manual chart reviews are inherently time-consuming and prone to human error, which can compromise data quality. To mitigate this risk, the hospital implemented several data validation techniques, including double-checking data entries, cross-referencing with pharmacy records for antibiotic administration, and conducting regular audits of the infection control database.

The hospital also established a data governance framework to standardize data collection procedures across departments. This included training staff on consistent documentation practices and creating a standardized checklist for chart reviews. These efforts helped ensure that the data used in quality measurement were accurate, complete, and consistent, ultimately leading to a 25% reduction in SSI rates over the course of the initiative.

Lessons Learned. This case study highlights the importance of rigorous data validation and governance in traditional quality measurement. Despite the manual nature of the data collection process, the hospital was able to achieve significant improvements in patient outcomes by prioritizing data quality and standardization. The success of this initiative underscores the value of careful planning and attention to detail in quality measurement efforts, even when using conventional data sources.

Case Study 2: Digital Quality Measurement in Chronic Disease Management

The second case study explores a digital quality measurement initiative implemented by a large healthcare system to improve chronic disease management. The system, which serves a diverse patient population across multiple states, sought to leverage digital tools to enhance the monitoring and management of patients with diabetes.

Data Collection and Integration. The healthcare system utilized EHRs, remote monitoring devices, and patient-reported outcomes (PROs) to collect data on key quality measures, such as blood glucose levels, medication adherence, and patient satisfaction. Data from wearable devices, such as continuous glucose monitors, were integrated into the EHR in real time, allowing providers to track patients' progress and intervene promptly if needed.

The system also employed machine learning algorithms to analyze the data and identify patterns that could predict adverse events, such as hypoglycemia or complications related to poor blood sugar control. These predictive analytic tools enabled proactive management of high-risk patients, improving overall outcomes.

Challenges and Solutions. One of the significant challenges in this digital measurement initiative was ensuring data interoperability across the various systems and devices used. The healthcare system had to overcome issues related to data standardization and integration, as different devices and EHR platforms used incompatible data formats. To address this, the system adopted the FHIR standard, which facilitated seamless data exchange and integration.

Another challenge was maintaining data privacy and security, particularly given the volume of sensitive health information being collected and transmitted across multiple platforms. The healthcare system implemented robust cybersecurity measures, including encryption, secure data transmission protocols, and regular security audits, to protect patient data.

Despite these challenges, the digital measurement initiative resulted in a 15% improvement in glycemic control among the system's diabetic patients and a significant reduction in emergency department visits related to diabetes complications.

Lessons Learned. This case study demonstrates the potential of digital measurement to enhance the quality of care in chronic disease management. By integrating real-time data from multiple sources and employing advanced analytics, the healthcare system was able to proactively manage patient care and achieve meaningful improvements in outcomes. However, the case also highlights the importance of addressing interoperability and security challenges to ensure the success of digital quality measurement initiatives.

Case Study Conclusions

These case studies underscore the importance of data quality, validation, and governance in both traditional and digital quality measurement efforts. While the methods and tools used may differ, the core principles of accurate, complete, timely, and consistent data remain essential to achieving meaningful improvements in healthcare quality. By learning from these real-world examples, healthcare organizations can better navigate the complexities of quality measurement and enhance their efforts to deliver high-quality care.

Future Directions

Healthcare data are evolving rapidly, and the increasing use of machine learning and artificial intelligence (AI) may challenge some of our traditional approaches to ensuring data validity. At the same time, these new technologies may create new opportunities for enhanced data collection. The recent emergence of large language models (LLMs), a type of AI built using machine learning techniques, natural language processing (NLP), and predictive modeling, is likely to be transformative for the healthcare data used in CQM [14, 15]. First, LLMs may be able to automate the population of standard data fields from unstructured data sources, including clinical notes and narratives. LLMs may in fact eliminate the need for standard data fields entirely, potentially reducing biases associated with predefined data priorities. Second, LLMs are particularly adept at summarizing data across various formats (i.e., notes, images, databases, devices) which could significantly improve both the quantity and quality of available data. Third, LLMs may shift the focus from retrospective CQMs to integrating quality directly into healthcare delivery, enhancing real-time patient care. However, it's essential to acknowledge potential drawbacks, including the risk of bias in LLM outputs, concerns about data privacy, and the possibility of over-reliance on automated systems that may overlook critical context. Each of these future directions represents an area of ongoing research, and the timeline for their impact remains uncertain. As we explore these advancements, it's crucial to consider complementary strategies that extend beyond LLMs to fully realize the potential of quality measurement in healthcare.

Discussion Questions

5.1 The chapter highlights accuracy, completeness, timeliness, and consistency as universal data requirements for quality measurement. Which of these challenges do you think poses the greatest barrier in healthcare today, and why? Can you think of real-world examples where these challenges impacted patient outcomes?

5.2 The adoption of standards like USCDI and FHIR aims to improve data capture and exchange. What are the potential benefits and drawbacks of these standards for healthcare providers, patients, and policymakers? How might these standards influence the scalability of quality measurement initiatives?

5.3 The chapter presents case studies contrasting traditional quality measurement with digital approaches. What are the trade-offs between these methods in terms of data validity, resource investment, and clinical impact? Which approach would you recommend for a small community hospital and why?

5.4 The chapter discusses the potential of LLMs and AI to transform quality measurement. How might these technologies improve data collection and analysis, and what ethical challenges (e.g., bias, privacy) do they present? How should healthcare systems address these concerns?

5.5 The chapter emphasizes the value of real-time data in facilitating continuous improvement and rapid intervention. What barriers exist to achieving real-time quality measurement across the healthcare system, and how could organizations overcome them? How might this shift impact patient care and provider workflows?

References

1 Define the Data Source(s). The Measures Management System. Centers for Medicare & Medicaid Services. https://mmshub.cms.gov/measure-lifecycle/measure-specification/define-data-sources (accessed 19 December 2024).

2 Liu, F. and Panagiotakos, D. (2022). Real-world data: a brief review of the methods, applications, challenges, and opportunities. *BMC Med. Res. Methodol.* 22 (1): 287. https://doi.org/10.1186/s12874-022-01768-6.

3 International Classification of Diseases, 10th Revision (ICD-10). ICD-10-CM Official Guidelines for Coding and Reporting. Centers for Disease Control and Prevention. https://www.cdc.gov/nchs/icd/icd-10-cm/index.html (accessed 19 December 2024).

4 D'Amore, J.D., Li, C., McCrary, L. et al. (2018). Using clinical data standards to measure quality: a new approach. *Appl. Clin. Inform.* 9 (2): 422–431. https://doi.org/10.1055/s-0038-1656548.

5 McClure, R.C., Macumber, C.L., Skapik, J.L., and Smith, A.M. (2020). Igniting harmonized digital clinical quality measurement through terminology, CQL, and FHIR. *Appl. Clin. Inform.* 11 (1): 23–33. https://doi.org/10.1055/s-0039-3402755.

6 United States Core Data for Interoperability (USCDI). Interoperability Standards Platform. HealthIT.gov (accessed 19 December 2024).

7 Fast Healthcare Interoperability Resources (FHIR) v5.0.0. HL7 International. https://hl7.org/fhir/ (accessed 19 December 2024).

8 Wang, Z., West, C.P., Vaa Stelling, B.E., et al. Measuring documentation burden in healthcare. Technical Brief No. 47. Agency for Healthcare Research and Quality; May 2024. AHRQ Publication No. 24-EHC023. https://doi.org/10.23970/AHRQEPCTB47.

9 Unified Medical Language System (UMLS). National Institutes of Health. https://www.nlm.nih.gov/research/umls/index.html (accessed 19 December 2024).

10 Value Set Authority Center. National Institutes of Health. https://vsac.nlm.nih.gov (accessed 19 December 2024).

11 U.S. Department of Health and Human Services. The HIPAA Privacy Rule. https://hhs.gov/hipaa/for-professionals (accessed 19 December 2024).

12 Trusted Exchange Framework and Common Agreement (TEFCA). https://www.healthit.gov/topic/interoperability/policy/trusted-exchange-framework-and-common-agreement-tefca (accessed 19 December 2024).

13 Certification of Health IT. https://www.healthit.gov/topic/certification-ehrs/certification-health-it (accessed 19 December 2024).

14 Li, Y., Wang, H., Yerebakan, H.Z., and Luo, Y. (2024). FHIR-GPT enhances health interoperability with large language models. *NEJM AI.* 1 (9): AIcs2300301.

15 Brat, G.A., Mandel, J.C., and McDermott, M.B.A. (2024). Do we need data standards in the era of large language models? *NEJM AI.* 1 (8): AIe2400548.

6

Measuring Cost and Efficiency in Healthcare

Taroon Amin¹, Jennifer Perloff², and Ashlie Wilbon Gyr³

¹Independent Consultant, New York, NY, USA

²Institute for Healthcare Systems, Brandeis University, Waltham, MA, USA

³Booz Allen Hamilton, Atlanta, GA, USA

Background

In 2021, healthcare expenditures accounted for nearly 20% of the US gross domestic product (GDP) [1]. At nearly $13,000, the United States spends more per person on healthcare than any other country. In comparison, Switzerland has the second highest spending at nearly $8,000 per person. In addition to total spending per person, the growth in healthcare spending is increasing at an alarming rate. Since 2020, there has been an increase in spending across multiple sites of care including hospitals, pharmacies, and clinician offices. This is accompanied by increases in healthcare insurance costs for Medicare, Medicaid, and commercial insurance with higher out-of-pocket costs for patients [1]. Understanding the drivers of these trends is a fundamental step toward identifying the most appropriate strategies for managing appropriate spending, utilization, and pricing.

Cost measures are a vital tool to help understand healthcare spending, including the relative allocation of resources to specific technologies, areas of healthcare, or populations of patients. Measuring cost gives us a lens into drivers of healthcare spending and serves as a tool that enables a standardized structure for measuring utilization across various settings and types of services. For convenience purposes, this chapter will use *cost measurement* to refer to both cost and resource use measurement. However, there are important distinctions between these two measurement approaches. Cost measures refer to measures that capture dollars paid to a provider (by the health plan, consumer, etc.) for services based on an established price, whereas resource use measures are designed to capture the absolute or relative investment of staff and supplies in the production of a given healthcare service based on a standardized unit (e.g., price, assigned value). Key components are the units of service (e.g., minutes of clinician time, number of X-rays) and the price per unit. This is often expressed in dollars (e.g., allowable charges, paid amounts, or standardized prices) [2].

Cost measures are different from quality measures. A quality measure typically refers to a structure, process, or outcome of care, while a cost measure focuses on the cost of producing that care. Structural and process measures are typically defined with a numerator and denominator and are typically reported in terms of percentages or rates. Similar to a quality outcome measure, cost measures are typically reported in terms of an observed-to-expected ratio whereby the numerator represents the observed or actual costs, and the denominator reflects expected costs. A ratio of 1 indicates that the cost is equal to the expected cost, and a ratio less than 1 indicates the actual cost is less than expected.

Approaches to Cost Measurement

There are two main approaches to defining a cost measure: per capita (e.g., cost per patient for a defined time period) or per episode (e.g., cost for an individual patient's clinical episode). Episode-based measures focus on aggregating costs accumulated for an episode of treatment specific to a condition (e.g., diabetes). Per capita measures count all costs for a specific timeframe, regardless of a clinical diagnosis (e.g., a measurement year). For per capita measures, typically the measurement window is time-based, for example, at the start of a measurement year. For episode-based measures, one needs to identify a trigger, such as Medicare diagnosis-related groups (DRGs), to signal a specific hospitalization, or an International Classification of Diseases, Tenth Revision (ICD-10), code, which would signal a specific diagnosis, to open an episode of care and start the counting of claims. Episode-based measures can be created as stand-alone measures or as groups of interrelated episodes in tools known as episode groupers. For example, an episode-based measure could capture the cost of an acute myocardial infarction (AMI), whereas an episode grouper may capture the cost of an AMI but also embed the cost of the AMI within a coronary artery disease (CAD) episode.

Other approaches to aggregate costs at the patient level can be used to determine per capita or per beneficiary costs for a defined time period, such as a measurement year. An example of this approach would be a total cost of care measure that includes all services associated with treating a patient including inpatient, outpatient, professional pharmacy, and ancillary services over a calendar year. Activity-based costing (ABC) is a less common, but notable, approach to measuring costs [3]. This approach enables providers to measure costs associated with care delivery processes (i.e., production costs).

For example, in the delivery of hip replacement surgery, each activity in the clinical process is monetized, including nursing labor, surgeon labor, and use of the operating room. ABC is less likely to be deployed as a standardized measure but can be a useful tool for providers to understand utilization and spending for cost drivers within a clinical setting.

Defining the Perspective

Many stakeholders incur costs as a part of a care delivery continuum. It is imperative to know whether the spending incurred is measured from the perspective of the consumer/patient, the health plan/payer, or the provider (e.g., hospital, clinic). Perspective has implications not only for the user to accurately interpret the results but also for a measure developer to identify data sources to provide accurate utilization counts and to determine how to count costs. For example, measuring costs from the perspective of a patient might focus on out-of-pocket costs (e.g., insurance premiums, co-pays). Therefore, the data source used to specify the measure should enable clear identification of the patient's utilization and spending. Measuring costs to the health plan typically involves counting claims billed to the insurer and assigning prices to those claims that the health plan has agreed to pay for each unit of service. Due to a significant variation in the amounts each health plan contracts to pay clinicians or hospitals, this approach to measuring actual prices paid is an important tool for understanding regional variation in costs. This approach, however, may not enable a comparison of utilization in different regions that provide the same services. This is because providers in different regions may charge different prices for the same services based on negotiated prices with commercial health plans. In order to facilitate comparisons of utilization, the counts of utilization must be monetized with standardized prices. These standard prices are determined for each type of service counted in the measure; all users of the measures apply the same set of standard prices for each service, regardless of region or contracted health plan prices. This standardized pricing methodology is generally used across measures developed by the Center for Medicare and Medicaid Services (CMS), including the total per capita cost measure and the Medicare Spending Per Beneficiary (MSPB) measures.

Context is key for interpreting cost measures. Since there is variation in the methodologies, data, and purposes of measuring cost, it is important to make transparent the intent of the measure and how analyzing variation in cost is consistent with that intent. Measure development or selection starts with a clear picture of the provider or entity responsible for the care delivered for an episode or a population. It is also important to define the goals of measurement, such as identifying areas of unnecessary utilization to achieve equal quality outcomes or examining differences in regional pricing. The specific context in which the measure is used will help ground measure design considerations. Similarly, for clinical episodes, the assignment of cost to the measure should be aligned with the purpose. Very inclusive assignments, such as all costs over a 90-day window or over a measurement year, are designed to identify variations in care patterns that may result in higher or lower costs. For example, a risk-adjusted total per capita cost measure can help to identify patterns of high-cost utilization, such as excess rates of acute hospitalizations or readmissions that care drive increased per capita spending within an attributed population of patients.

Designing Cost Measures

There are important interwoven considerations for designing a cost measure. These considerations are discussed in the context of the measure components and four overarching measure evaluation criteria, including importance to measure and report, scientific acceptability of the measure properties, usability, and feasibility. Measure components and the related considerations will be explored individually below.

Considerations

Table 6.1 summarizes the key interwoven considerations for designing cost measures. The amount and types of costs aggregated during the measurement period are impacted by how the time period is defined or type of utilization captured, for example, excluding costs related to medications for an asthma episode, where prescription medications are a key element of preventive treatment can give the impression that the costs associated with the asthma episode were much lower than actually spent. It is important to also recognize how environmental and systemic issues, such as access, may impact the results. In some cases, providers that deliver care to underserved populations may appear to have lower costs compared to others, but in fact, the lower costs may be due to lower utilization by a population that lacks access to appropriate care. Alignment of the intent of the measure and the scope of costs is important, and this includes timeframe, relationship with the measure topic, and services included.

Importance

Cost measures should capture a high-impact aspect of healthcare. High impact can be demonstrated by the number of individuals, the overall cost, substantial variation in cost, or cost performance that is consistently different from a target or benchmark for a subset of entities. For example, CMS uses the Medicare Spending per Beneficiary (MSPB) measure on the Care Compare website to show hospital cost performance compared to a national

Table 6.1: Key considerations for specifying cost measures.

Measure component	Key considerations
Measure type	The two most common cost measure types are per capita and episode-based measures. Episode-based measures are typically based on clinical condition, while per capita measures tend to focus on a specific timeframe (e.g., one year)
Time period	Selecting the time frame for a cost measure is a foundational step in establishing a measurement approach. It is intrinsically linked to the measure type and has implications for the scope of costs that will be captured in the measure
Risk adjustment	Risk adjustment is a tool used to account or control for clinical factors among the patient population and to balance the distribution of risk across the population. Consideration should be given to the purpose of risk adjustment in the context of the measure
Costing approach	Selecting a costing approach has implications for the interpretation of the results and the data needed to calculate the measure. Options include: ■ Actual prices paid by a health plan ■ Standardized prices ■ Relative value units (RVUs) ■ Prices billed to and paid by the patient (i.e., out-of-pocket costs)
Target population	The population targeted by the measure will drive measurement and testing decisions including which data sources should be used to calculate the measure and ensuring that the data set on which the measure is tested is representative of the target population to demonstrate validity and reliability in its intended context. Examples may include Medicare beneficiaries, all patients aged 18 years and older
Level of analysis	The level of analyses for which the measure is designed will determine the smallest unit to which the measure results can reliability be calculated and reported. For example, aggregating and reporting costs at the physician, hospital/provider, or health plan level may require different approaches to testing. Additionally, lower levels of analyses may have attribution challenges depending on the data source

average and a state average benchmark. Population-based cost measures tend to have more variation than episode-based measures because they tend to include a larger patient cohort that utilizes a broader range of clinical services. Further, consider existing cost measures to understand how the new cost measurement approach is an improvement from current measures.

Scientific Acceptability of Cost Measure Specifications

There are important considerations to ensure the measure specifications are reliable and valid. The specifications for a cost measure include the data protocol, clinical logic, construction logic, and adjustments for comparability. The adjustments for comparability include the approach to exclusions, risk adjustment, measure costing, and the attribution approach.

Data Protocol

All cost measures, whether they focus on the total cost of care or a specific clinical episode, require input data with information on cost. One common starting point is administrative data, including Medicare, Medicaid, and commercial paid claims from institutional and clinical providers. Additional data sources may include prescription drug data, durable medical equipment, and non-billable social services. Over time, new sources of cost information may become available and should be considered in the context of the measure intent.

For cost measures that utilize administrative claims data, reliability and validity require an understanding of the billing process, including the selection of services and diagnoses that are covered. For example, it is possible that in some regions there are strong incentives to record as many diagnoses as possible (e.g., high Medicare advantage penetration in a market), but in other regions, diagnostic coding is less intense. For episode measures, this variation in diagnostic coding can affect the number of cases that are opened. Other important data issues include missing data, beneficiary eligibility, and health insurance benefit design. In terms of missingness, many administrative claims data elements are not involved in payment, such as discharge disposition codes or location codes, and as a result may be left blank. In terms of eligibility, it is important to remember that individuals may frequently switch insurance plans and, as a result, may only be present in part of the data. For the individuals that switch plans, their total cost of care or episode-based cost of care may appear low due to the missing data. Many measure developers will require continuous coverage during the period of interest (e.g., a full year). This helps address the missing data problem but introduces other selection bias concerns. Specifically, are the individuals who switch plans similar to those individuals who are continuously enrolled?

Finally, insurance plan design is complex and some clinical services may not be covered. This can be very subtle, such as not reimbursing certain services billed by a nurse practitioner, or more obvious, like no coverage for dental care. All of these factors affect the accuracy and consistency of claims-based measures over time. Importantly, behavioral/mental health services or coverage may be outsourced (i.e., carved out) to specialty service providers and therefore completely missing in the medical claims data. It is important to take any outsourced services into account to ensure a valid comparison of utilization across payers.

Clinical Logic

All cost measures have some type of explicit or implicit clinical logic that helps determine what costs are included in the measure. The clinical logic for a cost measure defines the condition of interest and how that condition will be defined using diagnoses and procedures. The clinical logic for a measure should take into account comorbid conditions, disease interactions, clinical hierarchies, and clinical severity levels. In the case of episodes, the clinical logic can be complicated and require trigger codes to open an episode, rules to assign services to the episode, and, in some cases, exclusions. The "completeness" of the specification is important – cost measures that are too narrow may not be actionable. In other words, narrowly defined measures may not be informative about how to improve efficiency over time. For example, a cost measure of AMI hospitalization will have a narrow distribution of cost performance since it largely captures the DRG-based payment associated with the AMI. A broader measure may capture the AMI hospitalization and the 30 days post-discharge to assess the quality of the patient transition, including care coordination, post-acute care placement, and readmissions. On the other hand, per capita cost measures that are too broad may be hard for any one clinician to impact on his or her own. Per capita cost measures may also have clinical logic, such are excluding discretionary services like cosmetic surgery. These exclusions may be necessary as they are not a reflection of provider performance, but rather patient preferences. Ultimately, the clinical logic of the cost measure should be aligned with the measure intent.

Construction Logic

The construction logic specification for cost measures defines how the clinical logic can be applied to the underlying data used to calculate the measure. Measure specifications need to account for differences in how clinical services are captured and billed to Medicare, Medicaid, or commercial payers. These differences result in variations in the underlying administrative claims data used to calculate cost measures.

Adjustments for Comparability

Exclusions In both per capita cost of care and episode-based measures, services may be excluded based on the intent of the measure, the attribution model, and the accountable entity. For example, in the CMS Bundle Payment for Care Improvement (BPCI) program, car accidents and rare cancers were excluded because they are random, costly events that are often not directly preventable or directly related to actions taken by a clinician. However, services can be excluded to encourage the use of that service. For example, in a behavioral health episode cost measures focusing on depression, electroconvulsive therapy (ECT) may be excluded from the measure if payers and providers agree it is a service they want to encourage. Since

ECT is expensive, providers striving to be efficient may naturally look to minimize the use of the service if it were part of the episode cost measure. This type of inclusion or exclusion decision is a very powerful way to shape the incentives in episode-based measurement and highlights the importance of having stakeholders involved in the design.

Excluding services and excluding cases are often used to reduce variation in the observed costs. This is very important for making fair comparisons between providers or entities but also narrows the aperture of the measurement window, eliminating many opportunities to reduce the use of unnecessary services and improve efficiency. This trade-off between provider specificity (i.e., the services a given clinician bills) and systems opportunity (e.g., missed hand-offs between settings or other opportunities to improve efficiency) is a fundamental tension in the design of all cost measures.

Risk Adjustment   The purpose of risk adjustment is to take into account differences in patient severity between providers, organizations, or communities to make accurate relative inferences about the utilization, costs of care, and provider performance. Most measures use diagnostic information available in claims data to adjust cost measures, although some developers are beginning to experiment with electronic health record and registry data elements. All risk adjustment variables require careful consideration of timing, the use of information from discretionary versus non-discretionary services, and the precision of the risk model. As a rule, clinical risk factors should reflect a patient's health before he or she incurs cost. In practical terms, this means the creation of look-back windows (e.g., 6 or 12 months) to gather risk factors. There are concurrent risk adjustment models, such as the high-need risk model for dual eligible special needs plans, but these can conflate the timing of when a diagnosis occurs versus when costs occur. It can be controversial to include the use of specific services in a risk model because these are often done at the discretion of a provider. For example, if hospital admission is used as a risk adjustment variable for a pneumonia episode, the model may indirectly encourage clinicians to admit patients to the hospital. However, non-discretionary services, such as the use of a bypass machine during coronary artery bypass graft (CABG) surgery, can be a clever way to identify subtle clinical differences in patient populations using administrative data. Using a marker for the use of a bypass machine can help segment the patient population into different clinical risk categories in a way that cannot be done using diagnosis codes alone. Finally, model precision is critical. The less precise the risk model, the less protection it provides to clinicians or institutions who are being judged by measure performance or are taking on risk for the cost of care. Another risk protection that can be built into a cost measure is Winsorization, where costs are "capped" at a pre-defined threshold such as the 95th or 99th percentile. This technique helps to protect against the disproportional impact of high-cost outliers.

Attribution   Essential to all cost measures is a method of connecting the cost of care to the providers accountable for generating those costs. This is done through an attribution method that seeks to identify "accountable" entities by looking at who provides the bulk of a patient's care. The most common method is single attribution, where an individual clinician or healthcare entity (e.g., hospital or insurance plan) is assigned a measure based on the plurality or preponderance of a patient's care. This can lead to an episode of care being attributed to a clinician who feels like he or she does not have much influence over the patient's experience. However, it is important to understand the entire care team involved in generating costs. More advanced attribution models identify a primary care provider, a surgeon, a medical specialist, or the whole care team.

Disparities

All measures based on claims and encounters reflect the way care is delivered today. This means healthcare disparities, such as an AMI at an earlier age or limited prenatal care among Black and Latinx beneficiaries, will also be reflected in these measures. As a result, it is very important to think carefully about how historic lack of access or differential quality by race/ethnicity, disability status, region, or other factors is reflected in a cost measure that uses administrative data. Measure developers have many tools to address disparities, including the use of social determinants of health or area factors when developing an expected cost for a given group of beneficiaries. It is important to be intentional with this aspect of measure design and testing.

Measure Testing

When it comes to testing the reliability of a total cost of care or episode-based cost measure, developers may draw on a standard technique, such as split sample reliability, repeating the measure calculation in two randomly selected halves of the data or multiple years. It is important to think carefully about when and how a cost measure is supposed to vary over time when designing this type of test. For example, is it fair to assume the cost of a knee replacement episode is stable over multiple years? If not, it is likely not appropriate to examine spilt sample reliability over multiple years as a test of reliability. Rather, measuring correlation of accountable entity performance for two random samples within a year may be more appropriate in this case.

Conceptually, validity testing of a cost measure can be done by examining the correlation between the cost measure score results with other valid indicators of cost. Validity testing can also be conducted by examining performance among subgroups with known variation in cost. However, operationally, validity testing of cost measures is challenging. Typically, there are limited external cost data beyond administrative claims data to validate a cost measure against. Measure developers have relied on a limited sample of audited administrative claims data as evidence of data element validity, but this does not test the validity of the cost measure score. The area of validity testing for cost measures that are operationally feasible is underdeveloped.

Usability and Use

A goal of performance measurement is to ensure the intended audience of the measure can understand the results and find the results useful for decision-making. In the context of cost measurement, the intended audience may include patients and consumers and purchasers of health benefits, such as self-insured employers, health plans, and health plan participants. Given this range in the intended audience, it is important that cost performance is reported in the context of quality to facilitate the interpretability of performance results.

Cost measures should be transparent. This means clear specifications including the data protocol, clinical and construction logic, and adjustments for comparability. These methods individually, and when applied together, can be challenging to deconstruct. However, transparency can assist accountable entities in identifying how and where there are opportunities to improve cost performance.

Feasibility

The design of a cost measure needs to consider the extent to which the measure can be implemented without undue burden for the measure implementers and the accountable entities being measured. The current state of cost measurement primarily relies on administrative claims data that are routinely generated during the provision of care and in defined fields in electronic claims.

The feasibility of a cost measure should consider operational challenges. This field of measurement often includes complex measure methodologies, which in turn can limit the interpretability of the measure results. Further, complexity in the measure methodology can lead to errors in the coding of the measure. Also, given the use of administrative claims to implement most cost measure specifications, measure results can only be calculated at the close of the measurement period (i.e., adequate claims run out). This can limit the ability of the measures to inform care practices in real time.

Given the extensive use of cost measures in the private sector, and the use of commercial risk adjustment methodologies, those developing cost measures should consider how the use of proprietary components may impact the feasibility for those implementing the measure. These proprietary components may include value/code sets (e.g., current procedural terminology

(CPT) codes owned by the American Medical Association (AMA), risk adjustment models (e.g., Diagnostic Cost Group (DCG) or Adjusted Clinical Groups (ACG) models), or attribution algorithms. These proprietary components pose a challenge to accountable entities that may not have the resources to implement the measure, particularly those that require purchase and licensing.

Conclusion

With healthcare spending accounting for nearly 20% of the total US GDP, it is critical to have cost measures to assess cost drivers and identify opportunities for cost reduction. Cost measures can provide insight into pricing differences across regions, understanding which healthcare services, settings, or patient populations are driving spending. Broadly, cost measures provide a pathway to pinpoint where quality assessments should occur and where cost containment efforts for low-value care may need to be focused. However, when implemented as stand-alone measures, cost measures may lack directionality. It may not always be clear if higher or lower costs are "better" or "worse." For example, depending on the focus and timeframe, a short-term period of high costs may be expected in order to produce lower costs in the long term. Therefore, it is important to pair cost measures with quality measures. Provider report cards, price transparency websites, and other places where cost measures are used are most useful for consumer decision-making when they show which providers have the lowest cost for a given level of quality.

Discussion Questions

6.1 Why are cost measures essential in understanding healthcare spending, and how can they contribute to improving healthcare efficiency and resource allocation?

6.2 How do cost measures differ from quality measures in terms of their purpose, methodology, and implications for healthcare delivery?

6.3 What are the key challenges associated with developing and implementing cost measures, particularly regarding risk adjustment, attribution, and data feasibility?

6.4 Why is it important to pair cost measures with quality measures, and how can this pairing help identify potential unintended consequences in a meaningful way?

6.5 How does the perspective (e.g., patient, provider, or payer) influence the design and interpretation of cost measures, and what ethical considerations arise in choosing the perspective?

References

1 Center for Medicare and Medicaid Services. *National Health Expenditure Data Fact Sheet. CMS NHE Fact Sheet Website.* 2021. https://www.cms.gov/data-research/statistics-trends-and-reports/national-health-expenditure-data (accessed 1 December 2024).

2 National Quality Forum. *National Voluntary Consensus Standards for Cost and Resource Use: Technical Report April 2012.* 2012. https://www.qualityforum.org/WorkArea/linkit.aspx?LinkIdentifier=id&ItemID=70805 (accessed 1 December 2024).

3 Kaplan, R. and Porter, M. (2021). *The Big Idea: How to Solve the Cost Crisis in Health Care.* Harvard Business School Publishing.

4 National Quality Forum. *National Voluntary Consensus Standards for Cost and Resource Use: Final Report April 2021.* 2021. https://www.qualityforum.org/WorkArea/linkit.aspx?LinkIdentifier=id&ItemID=70788 (accessed 1 December 2024).

Appendix A. Cost Measurement Terms

The following cost measurement terms have been defined based on their use in the context of the chapter and adapted from consensus-based definitions [4].

Attribution – identifying and assigning a responsible provider or entity (e.g., health plan) for the care delivered for an episode or population.

Carve-outs – the outsourcing of services, such as behavioral health or pharmacy claims, to specialty health plans or claims processing entities or organizations.

Episode-grouper – automated tools often referred to as episode groupers are commonly used by commercial payers to parse and assign claims to clinical episodes using a complex set of rules based on hierarchies. These hierarchical rules identify the preferred clinical episode to which a claim should be assigned based on its relationship with the condition.

Exclusion criteria – criteria applied before a measure is tested in order to remove any individuals with conditions that may skew the final measure score.

Per capita measure – counts all services provided to a person within a specific population, regardless of condition or encounters with the system.

Per episode measure – counts resources based on bundles of services that are part of a distinctive event provided by one or multiple entities (e.g., health services provided associated with an event or series of events for acute myocardial infarction).

Risk adjustment – a corrective approach designed to reduce any negative or positive consequences associated with caring for patients of higher or lower health risk or propensity to require health services.

Standardized pricing – pre-established uniform price for a service, typically based on historical price, replacement cost, or an analysis of completion in the market; removes variation in resource costs due to differences in negotiated prices or geographic differences based on labor or other input costs.

7 Patient Safety Measurement

Edward J. Septimus

Department of Population Medicine, Harvard Pilgrim Healthcare, Boston, MA, USA

Introduction

Measuring patient safety and care quality as a means to promote improvement in care delivery is a national priority [1]. Over the last two decades, patient safety measurements have evolved and importance of patient safety has increased. By measuring patient safety and quality, we help identify gaps in care that can guide health system efforts to improve the delivery of safe and effective care and implement best practices. The goal of the cycle of quality improvement is to improve patient outcomes, ultimately lowering the rate of preventable adverse events (AEs) that reach patients. Efforts at advancing patient safety are guided by the idea that "you can't improve what you don't measure" [1]. Without measurement and transparency, clinicians, institutions, patients, and society cannot readily evaluate how the healthcare system is performing. It also cannot recognize that performance varies between and across health systems and among clinicians. This chapter briefly reviews the history of patient safety measurement and examples of how patient safety measurement has impacted clinicians, healthcare organizations, and policy. It concludes with a commentary on how patient safety measurements may change in the future.

History of Patient Safety Measures

Before the 1990s, patient safety was not a well defined concept in healthcare. While there were isolated efforts to track complications or AEs, these were often limited to specific procedures, departments, or conditions. In 1966, Avedis Donabedian developed a model that would later serve as the framework for assessing the quality and safety of healthcare by examining the relationship between three essential domains: structure (i.e., how is

Quality Measurement in Healthcare, First Edition. Edited by Jesse M. Pines, Helen Burstin, and Jane Hyatt Thorpe.
© 2025 Jesse M. Pines, Helen Burstin, and Jane Hyatt Thorpe.
Published 2025 by John Wiley & Sons Ltd.

healthcare designed), process (i.e., what care is delivered), and outcome (i.e., what happens to the patient) [2].

Researchers also began to utilize medical record to identify root causes of common quality care challenges, including the upswing in malpractice claims brought against clinicians. For example, the Harvard Medical Practice Study examined the incidence of AEs – defined as injuries caused by medical management – and the proportion of AEs that resulted from negligent or substandard care among hospitalized patients [3, 4]. They reported an AE rate of 3.7 events per 100 admissions. Twenty-eight percent of the AEs were judged to be caused by negligence, of which 15% led to death or permanent disability.

In 1998, the Advisory Commission on Consumer Protection and Quality in the Health Care Industry was established. A year later, the report from the Institute of Medicine (IOM), "To Err Is Human: Building a Safer Health System," was released [5]. The report, which estimated that between 44,000 and 98,000 Americans die each year due to medical errors, was a national wake-up call. Armed with the knowledge that medical errors were one of the leading causes of death in the United States, the Agency of Healthcare Research and Quality (AHRQ) developed patient safety indicators (PSIs) to identify potential in-hospital AEs from discharge data using the diagnoses on insurance claims. One such PSI is the rate of retained surgical items accidently left in patients during surgery, clearly an avoidable AE. Such events can be detected using insurance claims and can be used to measure the rate of these events within a hospital. Ideally the rate of this should be zero. In addition, the Joint Commission (TJC), which accredits hospitals, introduced National Patient Safety Goals. These were major efforts on the part of both public and private payers to drive patient safety starting with mandating measurement and reporting.

In the late 1990s and early 2000s, TJC launched its ORYX® initiative, the first national program for measuring hospital quality. Initially, ORYX® required the reporting only of non-standardized data on performance measures. In 2002, accredited hospitals were required to collect and report data on performance for at least two of four core measure sets (acute myocardial infarction, heart failure, pneumonia, and pregnancy). These data were made publicly available by TJC in 2004 [6]. The ORYX® initiative also required accredited organizations to collect and submit healthcare performance data to TJC on a continuous basis. In turn, TJC evaluated the data and used the performance information as part of an integrated accreditation process.

By introducing a data-driven and more continuous accreditation process, TJC increased the relevance and value of accreditation while supporting accredited organizations' internal quality improvement efforts. This was a significant advancement. At the time, few hospitals were using national data on quality measures to improve clinical care. Some hospitals strongly resisted collecting data on quality measures and reporting them publicly. This was due to concerns about misclassification and concerns that hospitals did not want to risk being publicly held accountable for their outcomes. There was also concern that application of measures in payment policies could have adverse effects on hospitals' finances and may not precisely discriminate differences in quality.

Despite these concerns, the promotion of public reporting and pay-for-performance has grown. In 2008, Medicare stopped reimbursing hospitals for treating eight preventable hospital-acquired conditions (HACs) such as falls, pressure ulcers, and certain infections [7]. Reduced payment is a strong incentive. This has driven hospital efforts toward preventing these conditions by improving the quality of care and implementing best practices, such as better infection control and nursing protocols. Beginning in 2012, the Centers for Medicaid & Medicare Services (CMS) Hospital Inpatient Value-Based Purchasing (VBP) Program took effect. VBP aimed to incentivize inpatient providers to deliver high value, as opposed to high-volume care. Payments are based on an acute care hospital's ability to meet performance measurements in six care domains: (1) patient safety; (2) care coordination; (3) clinical processes and outcomes; (4) population or community health; (5) efficiency and cost reduction; and (6) patient- and caregiver-centered experience. Under the program, CMS could withhold a percentage of Medicare payments as specified by law from poorly performing hospitals [8]. This form of payment holds healthcare providers accountable for both the cost and quality of care they provide. One example is a payment reduction of 1% for the worst-performing quartile under the Hospital Acquired Condition Reduction Program.

Criteria for Endorsing Quality and Safety Measures

When the Advisory Commission on Consumer Protection and Quality in the Health Care Industry was formed in 1997, the science of quality measurement was in its infancy. Measures were not widely available for many settings and conditions. The Commission recommended the establishment of two entities to provide leadership on improving quality and safety. The Advisory Council for Health Care Quality was envisioned as a governmental body responsible for (1) identifying national goals and objectives for quality measurement, improvement, and reporting and (2) tracking the nation's progress on goals and objectives in an annual report to the President and Congress. The second was the Forum for Health Care Quality Measurement and Reporting, which was a private body responsible for (1) implementing a comprehensive plan for measuring and reporting healthcare quality, (2) identifying core measures for standardized reporting, and (3) promoting development of core measures [9].

Out of this discussion, the Commission recommended the development of a public–private partnership to help standardize measures. Several organizations were already developing and evaluating quality and safety measures, and an even larger number of organizations started to collect measures to evaluate and report on the performance of providers. Public measure developers include CMS and the AHRQ, and non-profit private developers include TJC and the National Committee for Quality Assurance (NCQA).

In 1999, the National Quality Forum (NQF) was contracted by the US Department of Health and Human Services (HHS) in response to the Commission's work. From 1999 to 2023, the NQF served as a public–private partnership focused on setting standards for healthcare quality. NQF endorsed measures after a rigorous and transparent process and served as the consensus-based, standard-setting organization for quality and safety measures in the United States.

Using a rigorous evaluation and review process by multiple stakeholders, NQF-endorsed measures are considered the standard in measurement. Over the years, NQF has taken on a leadership role in measurement science and development, publishing expert and consensus reports on complex and controversial issues in measurement, including the adequacy of risk adjustment and strategies to link cost and quality. NQF reviews three general types of measures: (1) process measures that link a process to a desired outcome; (2) risk-adjusted outcome measures; and more recently, (3) electronic clinical quality measures (eCQMs). Over the years, NQF preferred outcome measures, and the proportion of outcome measures has consistently grown. The NQF has developed standard evaluation criteria for the endorsement of measures (Table 7.1) [10]. For each measure, the NQF required a rationale that supports

Table 7.1: National quality forum measure evaluation criteria.

1. Can the measure developer demonstrate the importance of the measure? *(must pass)*
   a. Does the evidence support the measure?
   b. Is there a performance gap, including disparities?

2. What is the scientific acceptability of the measure? *(must pass)*
   a. What is reliability and validity of measure?

3. Usability
   a. Can the measure be used for both accountability and performance improvement?
   b. Do the benefits to patients outweigh unintended consequences?

4. Feasibility
   a. Can data elements be routinely generated and used during routine care without undue burden?
   b. Can the data elements be captured in electronic health records (EHRs)?

the relationship between the outcome and at least one process, intervention, or service. Starting in 2023, the contract for consensus-based entity for quality measure assessment was moved to the contractor Batelle.

The American College of Physicians (ACP) has similar measure review criteria [11]. First, the evidence must demonstrate gaps in care, either considerable variation or suboptimal performance. The ACP calls this importance. Measure implementation should lead to measurable and meaningful improvement. Both organizations insist the evidence must be of high quality and represent best practices. They both recommend evaluating the measure specifications. Each measure must demonstrate both reliability and validity and distinguish good and poor quality. For outcome measures, risk adjustment should be adequately specified and valid. The goal is to use endorsed measures for decisions related to accountability and improvement. Therefore, each measure should also demonstrate usability. In essence, will the results provide information that will lead to improved care, and will it be publicly reported? Lastly, each measure should be feasible. Is it possible for the measure to be implemented without undue burden, and can the elements be captured electronically? Ultimately, these criteria are designed to vet the importance of a measure and determine whether it has the potential to drive improvement.

Beyond agency recommendations, expert guidance for establishing measurement endorsement criteria is available. In 2010, Chassin et al. published an article on how to use measurements to promote quality and safety [12]. Since process measures accounted for most measures at the time, they concentrated comments on accountability measures that address care processes. Despite the progress that had been made at the time, the authors felt there was room for improvement, particularly in using measures to optimize health benefits to patients. They proposed four criteria for measures that improve processes of care. First, a measure must be based on evidence that the process, when performed, leads to better outcomes. Second, the measure must accurately capture that the evidence-based care was delivered. Third, the measure must capture the process that approximates the desired outcome with relatively few intervening processes. Lastly, the measure should have minimal or no unintended consequences.

Chassin and colleagues provided a few examples of measures that were in use that did not meet their criteria. According to the criteria proposed by the authors, measures concerning smoking-cessation counseling and adults with acute myocardial infarction might fail to accurately capture the care process. Instead, those processes were only intended to "check the boxes" and did not result in better outcomes. For a process measure to be effective, it must link to better outcomes. A second example involved a measure calling for antibiotics to be given within four hours for patients admitted with suspected pneumonia. The authors were concerned that this measure had the potential to cause unintended consequences in patients ultimately not diagnosed as having pneumonia (i.e., unnecessary antibiotics to meet the measure). Such patients may then be at risk for antibiotic-related complications and delays in treatment of the actual diagnosis [13]. Because of documented unintended consequences, the measure was retired.

Practical Challenges with Safety Measurement and Reporting

Patient safety is a critical aspect of patient care that involves preventing harm or injury to patients while receiving medical care. Despite the growing interest in patient safety, recent studies highlight that harm resulting from medical care remains very common. In 2010, Landrigan and colleagues published a study of 10 North Carolina hospitals and found that harm and injury remained common, with little evidence of improvement despite substantial national attention and investment to improve the safety of care [14]. Another study in 2016 estimated that patient safety problems could lead to over 400,000 deaths per year and may be the third-leading cause of death in US hospitalized patients [15]. One must ask the question what does it mean to be safe? Is it a system of no errors or a system to minimize errors? Challenges include distinguishing safety from quality, as well as the negative connotation and punitive approaches around medical errors. The culture of shame and blame creates a toxic environment and discourages incident reporting. Safety improvement is also closely related to good management and effective implementation of a highly reliable culture of safety. A culture of safety is the foundation of safe and reliable care. It involves a systematic approach where safety principles are integrated into every aspect of the healthcare process, from administrative tasks to patient care practices where everyone is responsible for patient safety. This requires open transparent communication and a nonpunitive approach to reporting errors and near misses.

AEs can be detected either by observation or by claims which is not always reliable. One issue is presence on admission (e.g., a blood clot that the patient had when they were admitted to the hospital rather than one that occurred while in the hospital). Additionally, there may be lack of specificity about the cause. Since current approaches are also largely based on voluntary reporting, under-reporting of incidents is the norm with as few as 1% of incidents reported [16]. Other studies estimate that only 3–5% of AEs are reported [17, 18]. When reported, these events are sometimes investigated long after they occur, and recommendations for preventing future AEs may not always be implemented. However, incident reporting and analysis are critical for quality improvement efforts. An ideal system is one that captures AEs, when care harms patients, but also detects near misses, when errors occur without any harm [19]. Although many patient safety measures have been endorsed and are widely established (e.g., prevention of healthcare-associated infections

(HAIs)), many other patient safety domains lack good measures to track AEs and harm [20]. Table 7.2 lists some key patient safety measures.

This next section highlights the evolution of two safety domains to illustrate some of the issues raised: adverse drug events (ADEs) in hospitalized

Table 7.2: Key examples of patient safety measures.

1. Medication safety
   a. Medication reconciliation: accurately documenting and verifying a patient's medications at all care transitions
   b. Barcode scanning: using technology to match patients with their medications to prevent medication errors

2. Infection prevention
   a. Reduce CLABSIs, CAUTIs, SSIs, CDI, invasive MRSA
   b. Implementing the WHO Surgical Safety Checklist before surgical procedures
   c. Hand hygiene: regular and proper handwashing to prevent the spread of infections
   d. Proper sterilization and disinfection of medical equipment and surfaces
   e. Isolation precautions for patients with certain infectious diseases

3. Fall prevention
   a. Assessing patient's fall risk upon admission and implementing preventive measures to reduce falls

4. Communication and teamwork
   a. Encouraging open and effective communication among healthcare providers
   b. Promoting a culture of teamwork and collaboration
   c. Implementing tools like Situation, Background, Assessment, Recommendation (SBAR) for effective handoffs and communication to prevent miscommunications that can occur around care transitions

5. Adverse event reporting
   a. Encouraging a culture of reporting near misses and adverse events without fear of punishment
   b. Conducting root cause analysis to understand the causes of errors and prevent their recurrence
   c. Identifying adverse drug events

6. Healthcare technology
   a. Utilizing EHRs to improve documentation and access to patient information
   b. Employing technology (e.g., computerized provider order entry [CPOE]) to reduce medication errors

7. Patient experience
   a. Delivering patient-centered care

CLABSI, central line-associated bloodstream infection; CAUTI, catheter-associated urinary tract infection; SSI, surgical site infection; CDI, *Clostridioides difficile* infection; MRSA, methicillin-resistant *Staphylococcus aureus*; WHO, World Health Organization.

patients and HAIs, both of which are AEs. Here, we define an AE as "unintended physical injury resulting from or contributed to by medical care that requires additional monitoring, treatment, or hospitalization, or that results in death" [21]. AEs include both acts of omission (failure to diagnose) and acts of commission (incorrect diagnosis or treatment).

ADEs in Hospitalized Patients

Medication errors are one of the most common causes of harm [21, 22]. According to one report, 42% of life-threatening and serious ADEs were deemed preventable, compared with 18% of significant ADEs. Errors resulting in preventable ADEs occurred most often at the stages of ordering (56%) and administration (34%); transcription (6%) and dispensing errors (4%) were less common [22].

Over the last few decades, effective interventions have been developed to address ADEs. Specifically, computerizing the ordering of medications has reduced handwriting errors and delivering computerized clinical decision support has reduced the rate of serious drug interactions and administration of medications where patients have allergies [23, 24]. Another intervention, the barcoding of patients and medications, has reduced the rate of the wrong patients getting treated with a medication intended for another patient.

While some ADEs that occur may be immediately obvious such as when a patient is given medication where they have a known allergy, and it causes an immediate, serious allergic reaction. But the voluntary reporting of ADEs may miss a significant number of events, where the effect may be delayed or more subtle. For example, prescribing a non-steroidal anti-inflammatory medication at high doses may worsen kidney function, particularly for patients with prior kidney disease or other risk factors, but this effect may be delayed. The concern about the under-detection of ADEs has prompted research into better approaches to better assess medication safety. For instance, the Institute of Healthcare Improvement (IHI) developed the Global Trigger Tool (GTT) [25]. The GTT involves a chart review of discharge codes and summaries, medications, lab results, nursing notes, physician progress notes, and other comments to determine whether there is a "trigger" that might indicate an ADE. A trigger could be, for example, an order for an antihistamine in the case of allergic reaction, a medication stop order which could indicate an incorrect medication was ordered, or an abnormal lab result that could have been caused by a medication. The chart is then reviewed to see whether an ADE occurred and how severe it was. Classen et al. compared three methods to detect ADEs in hospitalized patients [26]. They found voluntary reporting and AHRQ Patent Safety Indicators missed 90% of ADEs, while the GTT found ten times more confirmed ADEs. The GTT has revealed uncounted events, especially ADEs. Although the GTT does a good job at identifying potential ADEs and is less resource-intensive than traditional record review, it still requires some resource commitment. In addition, the interrater reliability is low [14, 27]. Interrater reliability refers to the extent to which two or more individuals agree. GTT was not designed to identify every ADE. Unfortunately, the use of GTT to improve patient safety has resulted in little improvement overall [14, 28].

HAIs

Unlike measures for ADEs, there are established reliable measures for HAIs. HAI measurement and reporting have also evolved significantly over the last two decades. The Centers for Disease Control and Prevention (CDC) has created a valid and reliable measurement system through the National Healthcare Safety Network (NHSN). CDC has published standard surveillance definitions for central-line-associated bloodstream infections (CLABSIs), catheter-associated urinary tract infections (CAUTIs), *Clostridioides difficile* infections (CDIs), which can be caused by antibiotic use, methicillin-resistant *Staphylococcus aureus* (MRSA) bacteremia, and select surgical site infections (SSIs).

The CDC has also developed a risk-adjusted measure called standard infection ratio (SIR) which allows facilities to compare rates across different types of units. The SIR is calculated by dividing the number of observed infections by the number of predicted infections. The number of predicted infections is calculated using multivariable regression models that use multiple factors (e.g., patient age and comorbidities) generated from nationally aggregated data during a baseline period. This is compared to the number of actual infections that occur. A ratio of 1 means that the number of observed infections is what would have been expected. A ratio above 1, particularly when it is substantially above 1, means that more infections are occurring than expected and that interventions are needed to reduce the infection rate, such as implementing evidence-based practices (e.g., handwashing or sterile techniques for central line insertion). This approach to measurement is a valid way to assess infection rates over time and has been instrumental in driving down HAI rates over the past decade up until the pandemic.

Nationally, from 2015 to 2019, there have been consistent, significant reductions in the SIR for CLABSIs, CAUTIs, and CDI laboratory-identified (LabID), CDI, MRSA bacteremia, and SSIs [29]. Yet, despite significant improvement, HAIs are still a leading cause of preventable harm in US hospitals. Prevention of HAIs has remained a national priority as it is estimated that HAIs impact 1 of every 31 inpatients and leads to almost 30 billion in additional costs per year [30]. In a recent paper on the safety of inpatient care, the investigators reported on preventable AEs. Of the 978 AEs identified, 39% were ADEs, followed by events related to surgical or other procedures (30.4%), falls and pressure ulcers (15%), and HAIs (11.9%) [21]. Although substantial improvements had been made in reducing HAIs over the past decade, the COVID-19 pandemic led to a resurgence of almost all major HAIs [31]. Several factors have been identified to account for the reversal of the prior improvements in this area. This includes a diversion of infection prevention resources to COVID-19 response, staffing challenges and shortage of personnel protective equipment [32]. Nonetheless, the high ongoing burden of HAIs is particularly tragic given that over 50% may be preventable with proper infection prevention, control, and patient safety interventions [33].

Future Directions in Patient Safety Measurement

Currently, our ability to measure patient safety in a reliable, effective, and timely way remains limited. Many facilities still rely on voluntary reporting, manual chart review, or post-discharge coding to capture AEs. Identifying AE in electronic health records (EHRs) using computerization of electronic detection of triggers with or without artificial intelligence (AI) is the future. This has led to a significant number of eCQMs, which have been recently endorsed to measure AEs. eCQMs are standardized performance measures in an electronic format and promote greater consistency in measure development and in measuring and comparing performance results. They also can provide more exact requirements about where information should be collected and drive greater standardization across the measures and greater confidence in comparing outcomes and provider performance. The Health Information Technology for Economics and Clinical Health (HITECH) Act provided guidelines for a nationwide technology infrastructure. A key element of the Act is to use eCQMs [34]. In the future, the use of EHRs to collect and report quality measures will continue to grow and using electronic sources will continue to reduce the burden of reporting on measures.

Patient safety active management system (PSAM) is one example. Sammer et al. developed a novel automated all-cause harm trigger identification PSAM that allowed for real-time bedside intervention, real-time trend analysis affecting patient safety, and continued learning about harm measurement. PSAM generates a patient safety predictive score from real-time data from the EHR. In the study, the organization applied algorithms which in turn generated triggers or potential AEs. A nurse reviewer would then follow the electronic triggers to determine whether patient harm occurred [35]. The automated harm trigger system revealed not only a higher rate of harm but a broader scope (e.g., different harm types). This led to a deeper understanding of patient safety vulnerabilities and how to address them. In another study, investigators used the same PSAM system in two community hospitals. They confirmed that PSAM could not only detect harm in real time but at higher rates [36].

Two recent articles outline the potential applications of AI to improve patient safety. Both feel AI has significant potential to improve patient safety including AEs. The articles outline some limitations and the challenges in evaluating these systems [37, 38]. The authors urge caution, however, as evidence of the impact of AI on safety and outcomes is limited and conflicting. For example, one study reported that an automated predictive model to identify high-risk patients for whom interventions by rapid-response teams could be implemented was associated with decreased mortality [39]. In contrast, another study demonstrated a proprietary sepsis prediction model had poor discrimination and calibration in predicting the onset of sepsis [40]. For AI to be effective, implementation will require health systems to develop and rigorously validate AI in real-world settings. We will need to create a public–private partnership to critically evaluate AI and patient safety.

This same concept applies to HAI measurement. HAI surveillance is currently performed by infection preventionists. They currently review medical records and apply standard surveillance definitions for HAIs and then enter data into the NHSN database. This can be labor intensive, and definitions can be complicated leading to subjective interpretation. Currently, NHSN utilizes the Clinical Data Architecture (CDA) for electronic data transfer including MRSA bacteremia and laboratory-identified CDI. In 2024, NHSN will add healthcare onset antibiotic-treated CDI (HT-CDI), which will involve a combination of any positive test and treatment on or after day 4 from admission [41] and hospital-onset bacteremia (HOB) and fungemia to capture all potential device-related HOB besides CLABSI [42]. These are newly endorsed measures and will be fully captured electronically. This transition is consistent with CMS's plan to move to a digital platform [43].

Another approach being evaluated is the CDC's hospital-onset adult sepsis event (ASE) definition. This would entail using routine electronic clinical data to flag patients with concurrent clinical indicators of presumed serious infections (i.e., blood culture orders and sustained treatment with antibiotics) and concurrent organ dysfunction (i.e., initiation of vasopressors or mechanical ventilation or significant changes in laboratory values). Preliminary data suggest that the CDC's hospital-onset sepsis surveillance definition may identify many more HAIs than current CMS reportable metrics and that hospital-onset sepsis is associated with very high mortality rates even when current reportable HAIs are absent [44]. ASE surveillance could also increase the efficiency and clinical significance of surveillance while identifying new targets for prevention.

Conclusion

Despite progress in safety measurement and reporting and improvements in medication safety, much more needs to be done. Our ability to measure AEs reliably remains limited; however, innovations are being tested that may improve this ability in the future. Healthcare systems need to expand their patient safety infrastructure to address emerging safety opportunities and translate evidence into practice in a timely manner. Computerization of electronic detection of triggers with or without AI is the future. To improve patient safety, outcomes, and cost savings, consistent and reliable measures for reporting harm must be in place. Migrating to electronic quality measures will shift the burden from manual data collection to electronic systems. eCQMs will become the standard in assessing quality and outcomes in the future. While this chapter focused on inpatients, the same opportunities apply to outpatient measures and across the continuum of care.

Discussion Questions

7.1 Given the limitations of voluntary reporting and manual chart reviews in identifying AEs, how can healthcare systems balance the need for accurate data collection with the burden on providers?

7.2 How can advancements in EHRs and AI enhance the detection and reporting of AEs? What are the risks or challenges associated with implementing these technologies?

7.3 The "shame and blame" culture has been cited as a barrier to effective incident reporting. What steps can healthcare organizations take to foster a culture of safety and transparency?

7.4 How should healthcare organizations prioritize between process measures (e.g., handwashing compliance) and outcome measures (e.g., rates of hospital-acquired infections) to improve patient safety effectively?

7.5 As healthcare moves toward automated and eCQMs, what ethical considerations and safeguards should be put in place to ensure patient data privacy and the accuracy of automated systems?

References

1 Brook, R.H., McGlynn, E.A., and Cleary, P.D. (1996). Measuring quality of care. *N. Engl. J. Med.* 335 (13): 966–970. https://doi.org/10.1056/nejm199609263351311.

2 Donabedian, A. (2005). Evaluating the quality of medical care. 1966. *Milbank Q.* 83 (4): 691–729 (In English). https://doi.org/10.1111/j.1468-0009.2005.00397.x.

3 Brennan, T.A., Leape, L.L., Laird, N.M. et al. (1991). Incidence of adverse events and negligence in hospitalized patients. *N. Engl. J. Med.* 324 (6): 370–376. https://doi.org/10.1056/nejm199102073240604.

4 Leape, L.L., Brennan, T.A., Laird, N. et al. (1991). The nature of adverse events in hospitalized patients. *N. Engl. J. Med.* 324 (6): 377–384. https://doi.org/10.1056/nejm199102073240605.

5 Institute of Medicine (US) Committee on Quality of Health Care in America; Kohn, L.T., Corrigan, J.M., Donaldson, M.S. (eds.). (2000). *To Err is Human: Building a Safer Health System*. National Academy Press.

6 Lee, K.Y., Loeb, J.M., Nadzam, D.M., and Hanold, L.S. (2000). Special report: an overview of the joint commission's ORYX initiative and proposed statistical methods. *Health Serv. Outcomes Res. Methodol.* 1 (1): 63–73. https://doi.org/10.1023/A:1010010221434.

7 McNair, P.D., Luft, H.S., and Bindman, A.B. (2009). Medicare's policy not to pay for treating hospital-acquired conditions: the impact. *Health Aff.* 28 (5): 1485–1493 (In English). https://doi.org/10.1377/hlthaff.28.5.1485.

8 Blumenthal, D. and Jena, A.B. (2013). Hospital value-based purchasing. *J. Hosp. Med.* 8 (5): 271–277 (In English). https://doi.org/10.1002/jhm.2045.

9 McGlynn, E.A. (2003). Introduction and overview of the conceptual framework for a national quality measurement and reporting system. *Med. Care* 41 (1): I1–I7. http://www.jstor.org.srv-proxy2.library.tamu.edu/stable/3767723.

10 Burstin, H., Leatherman, S., and Goldmann, D. (2016). The evolution of healthcare quality measurement in the United States. *J. Intern. Med.* 279 (2): 154–159. https://doi.org/10.1111/joim.12471.

11 MacLean, C.H., Kerr, E.A., and Qaseem, A. (2018). Time out – Charting a path for improving performance measurement. *N. Engl. J. Med.* 378 (19): 1757–1761. https://doi.org/10.1056/NEJMp1802595.

12 Chassin, M.R., Loeb, J.M., Schmaltz, S.P., and Wachter, R.M. (2010). Accountability measures – Using measurement to promote quality improvement. *N. Engl. J. Med.* 363 (7): 683–688. https://doi.org/10.1056/NEJMsb1002320.

13 Metersky, M.L. (2008). Measuring the performance of performance measurement. *Arch. Intern. Med.* 168 (4): 347–348. https://doi.org/10.1001/archinternmed.2007.81.

14 Landrigan, C.P., Parry, G.J., Bones, C.B. et al. (2010). Temporal trends in rates of patient harm resulting from medical care. *N. Engl. J. Med.* 363 (22): 2124–2134. https://doi.org/10.1056/NEJMsa1004404.

15 Makary, M.A. and Daniel, M. (2016). Medical error—The third leading cause of death in the US. *BMJ* 353: i2139. https://doi.org/10.1136/bmj.i2139.

16 Wakefield, J.G. and Jorm, C.M. (2009). Patient safety – a balanced measurement framework. *Aust. Health Rev.* 33 (3): 382–389. https://doi.org/10.1071/AH090382.

17 Sari, A.B., Sheldon, T.A., Cracknell, A., and Turnbull, A. (2007). Sensitivity of routine system for reporting patient safety incidents in an NHS hospital: retrospective patient case note review. *BMJ* 334 (7584): 79 (In English). https://doi.org/10.1136/bmj.39031.507153.AE.

18 Classen, D. (2003). Medication safety: moving from illusion to reality. *JAMA* 289 (9): 1154–1156. https://doi.org/10.1001/jama.289.9.1154.

19 Clarke, J.R. (2006). How a system for reporting medical errors can and cannot improve patient safety. *Am. Surg.* 72 (11): 1088–1091; discussion 1126–1148 (In English). https://doi.org/10.1177/000313480607201118.

20 Bates, D.W. and Singh, H. (2018). Two decades since to err is human: an assessment of progress and emerging priorities in patient safety. *Health Aff.* 37 (11): 1736–1712 (In English). https://doi.org/10.1377/hlthaff.2018.0738.

21 Bates, D.W., Levine, D.M., Salmasian, H. et al. (2023). The safety of inpatient health care. *N. Engl. J. Med.* 388 (2): 142–153. https://doi.org/10.1056/NEJMsa2206117.

22 Bates, D.W., Cullen, D.J., Laird, N. et al. (1995). Incidence of adverse drug events and potential adverse drug events. Implications for prevention. ADE Prevention Study Group. *JAMA* 274 (1): 29–34 (In English).

23 Kaushal, R., Shojania, K.G., and Bates, D.W. (2003). Effects of computerized physician order entry and clinical decision support systems on medication safety: a systematic review. *Arch. Intern. Med.* 163 (12): 1409–1416 (In English). https://doi.org/10.1001/archinte.163.12.1409.

24 Prgomet, M., Li, L., Niazkhani, Z. et al. (2017). Impact of commercial computerized provider order entry (CPOE) and clinical decision support systems (CDSSs) on medication errors, length of stay, and mortality in intensive care units: a systematic review and meta-analysis. *J. Am. Med. Inform. Assoc.* 24 (2): 413–422 (In English). https://doi.org/10.1093/jamia/ocw145.

25 Classen, D.C., Lloyd, R.C., Provost, L. et al. (2008). Development and evaluation of the institute for healthcare improvement global trigger tool. *J. Patient Saf.* 4 (3): 169–177.

26 Classen, D.C., Resar, R., Griffin, F. et al. (2011). 'Global trigger tool' shows that adverse events in hospitals may be ten times greater than previously measured. *Health Aff.* 30 (4): 581–589 (In English).

27 Hanskamp-Sebregts, M., Zegers, M., Vincent, C. et al. (2016). Measurement of patient safety: a systematic review of the reliability and validity of adverse event detection with record review *BMJ Open* 6 (8): e011078 (In English). https://doi.org/10.1136/bmjopen-2016-011078.

28 Stockwell, D.C., Bisarya, H., Classen, D.C. et al. (2015). A trigger tool to detect harm in pediatric inpatient settings. *Pediatrics* 135 (6): 1036–1042 (In English). https://doi.org/10.1542/peds.2014-2152.

29 Dudeck, M., Edwards, J., Godfrey-Johnson, D. et al. (2020). Incidence trends of central-line–associated bloodstream infections in acute-care hospitals, NHSN, 2009–2018. *Infect. Control Hosp. Epidemiol.* 41 (S1): s294–s295. https://doi.org/10.1017/ice.2020.873.

30 Magill, S.S., O'Leary, E., Janelle, S.J. et al. (2018). Changes in prevalence of health care–Associated infections in U.S. Hospitals. *N. Engl. J. Med.* 379 (18): 1732–1744. https://doi.org/10.1056/NEJMoa1801550.

31 Weiner-Lastinger, L.M., Pattabiraman, V., Konnor, R.Y. et al. (2022). The impact of coronavirus disease 2019 (COVID-19) on healthcare-associated infections in 2020: a summary of data reported to the National Healthcare Safety Network. *Infect. Control Hosp. Epidemiol.* 43 (1): 12–25 (In English). https://doi.org/10.1017/ice.2021.362.

32 Bearman, G., Cooper, K., Doll, M. et al. (2020). Impact of COVID-19 on traditional healthcare-associated infection prevention efforts. *Infect. Control Hosp. Epidemiol.* 41 (8): 946–947. https://doi.org/10.1017/ice.2020.141.

33 Schreiber, P.W., Sax, H., Wolfensberger, A. et al. (2018). The preventable proportion of healthcare-associated infections 2005–2016: systematic review and meta-analysis. *Infect. Control Hosp. Epidemiol.* 39 (11): 1277–1295 (In English). https://doi.org/10.1017/ice.2018.183.

34 Blumenthal, D. and Tavenner, M. (2010). The "Meaningful Use" regulation for electronic health records. *N. Engl. J. Med.* 363 (6): 501–504. https://doi.org/10.1056/NEJMp1006114.

35 Sammer, C., Miller, S., Jones, C. et al. (2017). Developing and evaluating an automated all-cause harm trigger system. *Jt. Comm. J. Qual. Patient Saf.* 43 (4): 155–165 (In English). https://doi.org/10.1016/j.jcjq.2017.01.004.

36 Classen, D., Li, M., Miller, S., and Ladner, D. (2018). An electronic health record–based real-time analytics program for patient safety surveillance and improvement. *Health Aff.* 37 (11): 1805–1812 (In English). https://doi.org/10.1377/hlthaff.2018.0728.

37 Bates, D.W., Levine, D., Syrowatka, A. et al. (2021). The potential of artificial intelligence to improve patient safety: a scoping review. *NPJ Digit. Med.* 4 (1): 54 (In English). https://doi.org/10.1038/s41746-021-00423-6.

38 Classen, D.C., Longhurst, C., and Thomas, E.J. (2023). Bending the patient safety curve: how much can AI help? *NPJ Digit. Med.* 6 (1): 2 (In English). https://doi.org/10.1038/s41746-022-00731-5.

39 Escobar, G.J., Liu, V.X., Schuler, A. et al. (2020). Automated identification of adults at risk for in-hospital clinical deterioration. *N. Engl. J. Med.* 383 (20): 1951–1960. https://doi.org/10.1056/NEJMsa2001090.

40 Wong, A., Otles, E., Donnelly, J.P. et al. (2021). External validation of a widely implemented proprietary sepsis prediction model in hospitalized patients. *JAMA Intern. Med.* 181 (8): 1065–1070. https://doi.org/10.1001/jamainternmed.2021.2626.

41 Kociolek, L.K., Gerding, D.N., Carrico, R. et al. (2023). Strategies to prevent *Clostridioides difficile* infections in acute-care hospitals: 2022 update. *Infect. Control Hosp. Epidemiol.* 44 (4): 527–549. https://doi.org/10.1017/ice.2023.18.

42 Classen, D.C., Rhee, C., Dantes, R.B., and Benin, A.L. (2023). Healthcare-associated infections and conditions in the era of digital measurement. *Infect. Control Hosp. Epidemiol.* 1–6 (In English). https://doi.org/10.1017/ice.2023.139.

43 Schreiber, M., Krauss, D., Blake, B. et al. (2021). Balancing value and burden: the Centers for Medicare & Medicaid Services electronic Clinical Quality Measure (eCQM) Strategy Project. *J. Am. Med. Inform. Assoc.* 28 (11): 2475–2482 (In English). https://doi.org/10.1093/jamia/ocab013.

44 Page, B., Klompas, M., Chan, C. et al. (2021). Surveillance for healthcare-associated infections: hospital-onset adult sepsis events versus current reportable conditions. *Clin. Infect. Dis.* 73 (6): 1013–1019 (In English). https://doi.org/10.1093/cid/ciab217.

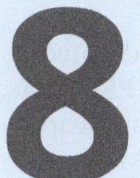

8 Patient-Reported Outcomes in Performance Measures

Margaret Morris[1], Patricia D. Franklin[1,2,3], Nan E. Rothrock[1,4,5], and David Cella[1,4,5]

[1]Department of Medical Social Sciences, Northwestern University Feinberg School of Medicine, Chicago, IL, USA

[2]Department of Orthopaedic Surgery, Northwestern University Feinberg School of Medicine, Chicago, IL, USA

[3]Department of Medicine, Northwestern University Feinberg School of Medicine, Chicago, IL, USA

[4]The Ken and Ruth Davee Department of Neurology, Northwestern University Feinberg School of Medicine, Chicago, IL, USA

[5]Department of Psychiatry and Behavioral Sciences, Northwestern University Feinberg School of Medicine, Chicago, IL, USA

Introduction

Patient-generated data are increasingly utilized by the Centers for Medicare & Medicaid Services (CMS) to measure healthcare quality [1–6]. With the implementation of patient-reported outcome performance measures (PRO-PMs), CMS intends to reward excellence and incentivize improvement, resulting in better healthcare driven by patients' treatment and outcome priorities [2].

Quality Measurement in Healthcare, First Edition. Edited by Jesse M. Pines, Helen Burstin, and Jane Hyatt Thorpe.
© 2025 Jesse M. Pines, Helen Burstin, and Jane Hyatt Thorpe.
Published 2025 by John Wiley & Sons Ltd.

This chapter provides a brief introduction to patient-reported outcome measures (PROMs), describes key aspects in the development of PRO-PMs, contrasts factors limiting current use with opportunities for potential application of PRO-PMs, and proposes future directions for PRO-PM creation and adoption.

Definitions

Central to this discussion is the relationship between PROs, PROMs, and PRO-PMs as illustrated in Figure 8.1. PROs are outcomes experienced by patients, and PROMs are instruments used to measure the outcomes. Quality is measured using PRO-PMs. Detailed definitions and examples are presented in Table 8.1.

Patient-Reported Outcome Measures

PROMs uniquely capture the voice of the patient in terms of the patient's perception of their health outcomes. PROMs measure a patient's symptoms, function, and well-being, using direct inquiry without interpretation by others. They assess many different aspects of health and can be classified into four categories defined in Table 8.2.

Of these four types of PROMs, the first three (health-related quality of life [HRQoL], functional status, and symptoms/symptom burden) are primarily used in PRO-PMs.

Key Concepts

Reliability and Validity

While this chapter does not include a rigorous discussion of the science behind PROM development, it is important to understand the basic psychometric concepts listed in Table 8.3 that are used in measure evaluation and testing.

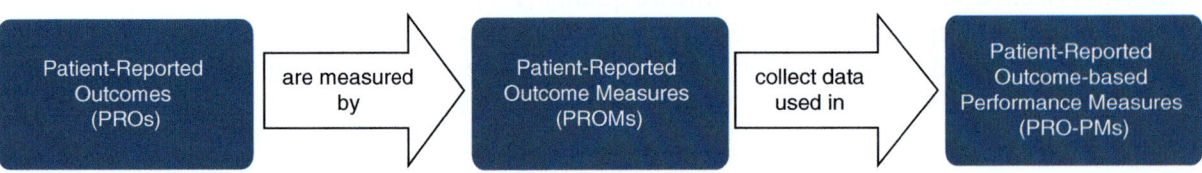

Figure 8.1: Relationship between PROs, PROMs, and PRO-PMs.

Table 8.1: Definitions.

Concept	Definition	Examples
Patient	"A person who is receiving healthcare services or using long-term healthcare support services" [1]	"Patient" may refer more broadly to include patient proxies such as parent of a pediatric patient
Patient-reported outcome (PRO)	"Any information on the outcomes of healthcare obtained directly from patients without modification by clinicians or other healthcare professionals" [1]	Depression Pain Anxiety
Patient-reported outcome measure (PROM)	"Any standardized or structured questionnaire regarding the status of a patient's health condition, health behavior, or experience with healthcare that comes directly from the patient (i.e., a PRO). The use of a structured, standardized tool such as a PROM will yield quantitative data that enables comparison of patient groups or providers" [1]	PHQ-9 PROMIS Depression, Physical Function, etc.
Performance measures	"A gauge used to assess the performance of a process or function of any organization. Quantitative or qualitative measures of the care and services delivered to enrollees (process) or the end result of that care and services (outcomes)" [7]	See PRO-PM example
Patient-reported outcome-based performance measure (PRO-PM)	"A performance measure that is based on patient-reported outcomes assessed through data often collected through a PROM and then aggregated for an accountable healthcare entity" [1]	Percentage of patients in an accountable care organization with an improved depression score as measured by PHQ-9

Table 8.2: Categories of PROs measured by PROMs.

PRO category	Definition
1. Health-related quality of life (HRQoL)	"A multidimensional [8] survey construct encompassing physical, social, and emotional well-being associated with illness and its treatment" [9]
2. Functional status	"Refers to a patient's ability to perform both basic and more advanced (instrumental) activities of daily life" [10]
3. Symptoms and symptom burden	Symptoms are manifestations of a disease that are apparent to the patient. "Symptom burden is defined as the subjective, quantifiable prevalence, frequency, and severity of symptoms placing a physiologic burden on patients and producing multiple negative, physical, and emotional patient responses" [11]
4. Health behaviors	"Actions taken by individuals that affect health or mortality. These actions may be intentional or unintentional, and can promote or detract from the health of the actor or others" [12] (e.g., smoking)

Table 8.3: Psychometric concept definitions.

Concept	Definition
Reliability	"The extent to which a scale or measure yields reproducible and consistent results" [13]
	"Reliability of *data elements* refers to repeatability and reproducibility of the data elements for the same population in the same time period. Reliability of the *measure score* refers to the proportion of variation in the performance scores attributable to systematic differences across the measured entities (or signal) in relation to the random error (or noise)" [1]
Validity	"The extent to which an instrument measures what it is intended to measure and can be useful for its intended purpose" [13]
	"Validity of *instruments* can be assessed in numerous ways, often in comparison with an authoritative source (such as a similar validated instrument). Validity of *measure scores* can refer to the correctness of conclusions that users might draw from a reliable and valid instrument (as, for instance, that a better score on a quality measure reflects higher quality of health care)" [1]

PROM Scoring

PROM scoring can be based on either *classical test theory*, which features a fixed set of questions and calculation of raw scores, or *item response theory (IRT)*, which also enables computer-adaptive tests (CATs) where future questions are tailored to the individual patient based on their previous responses. IRT offers advantages over classical testing theory [1]:

- Measures can be shorter, thereby reducing the patient burden.
- "Response pattern" scoring used with IRT-calibrated PROMs is more accurate than classical test theory scoring.

The growing use of IRT and associated CATs in healthcare is fueled by the NIH-sponsored PROMIS, which provides computer application programming interface (API) access to 1000+ validated measures [3]. Many PROMIS measures are available as CATs and as fixed short-form questionnaires [14], allowing clinicians the flexibility of initial short-form implementation transitioning to PROMIS CATs via the API. With a carefully designed implementation strategy, PROMIS CATs can effectively be integrated into the clinical workflow [15].

Patient-Reported Outcome-Based Performance Measurement

PRO-PM use in quality initiatives requires processes for the creation, endorsement, collection, analysis, and interpretation of clinically validated PROM data. Leveraging core quality measurement processes extended to address

PRO-PM-specific requirements has laid the groundwork for implementation in existing regulatory programs [4].

Building PRO-PMs

The development of PRO-PMs for accountability is a complex and multi-phased challenge requiring a precisely defined scientific process. The *CMS Measure Management System* (MMS) serves as a core quality measurement process, defined as "a standardized system for developing and maintaining the quality measures used in various CMS initiatives and programs" [16]. Supplemental guidance is provided to address special considerations in PRO-PM development [2]. Additionally, due to the complexity of PRO-PMs, technical guidance in the form of a roadmap was created to assist measure developers and serve as a catalyst for PRO-PM development [4].

Building the Roadmap

CMS, in partnership with the National Quality Forum (NQF), launched the *"Building a Roadmap from Patient-Reported Outcome Measures to Patient-Reported Outcome Performance Measures"* project in 2020 [4]. A multi-disciplinary technical expert panel was assembled for the project. CMS-commissioned manuscripts from 2012 to 2015 [1, 17, 18] served as the foundation for technical guidance in PRO-PM measure development. In November 2022 when the guidance was first introduced, PRO-PMs were under-represented across endorsed measures, comprising less than 7% of the total number of certified performance measures [4].

Roadmap Overview

The PRO-PM roadmap illustrated in Figure 8.2 outlines a process with seventeen tasks organized into four stages. Measures are promoted through each stage from initial definition of goals to final implementation and endorsement of the PRO-PM. Progression is flexible and iterative to allow for variation in the complexity and structure of proposed measures [4].

The four stages (and 17 tasks) in the roadmap are:

- **Stage 1:** Definition of measurement goals (six tasks)
- **Stage 2:** Exploration and assessment of PROMs (three tasks)
- **Stage 3:** Development and testing of the PRO-PM (six tasks)
- **Stage 4:** Finalization and implementation of the PRO-PM (two tasks)

This process aims to be patient-centered. Patients and patient advocates are included from project initiation through final implementation. Patient-driven measure goal definition encourages alignment of ensuing steps with patients' treatment and outcome priorities. As the focus of the process shifts toward PROM selection, factors such as *interpretability*, *feasibility*

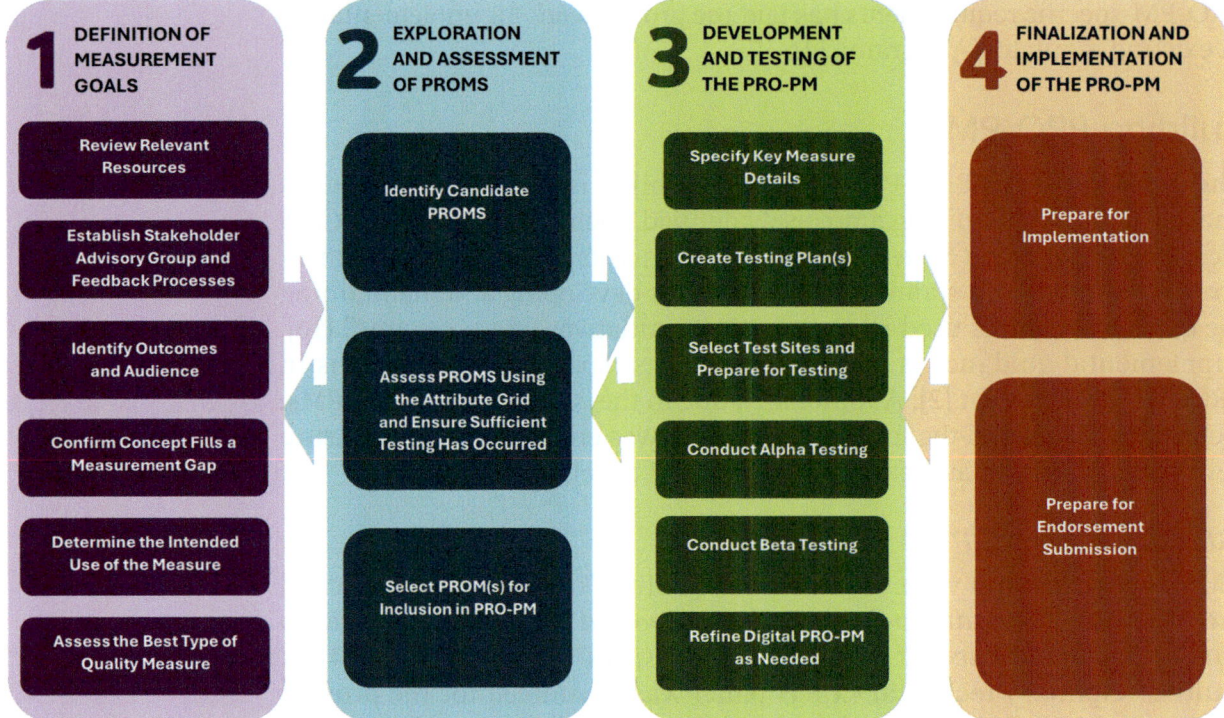

Figure 8.2: Overview of the National Quality Forum PRO-PM Roadmap.

Source: Reproduced from Ref. [4]/12/The National Quality Forum.

of integration into the clinical workflow, and *psychometric properties of PROMs* demand that clinician and psychometrician user requirements are also prioritized [4].

Selecting PROMs for PRO-PMs

NQF expanded on previous publications on the process for selecting PROMs appropriate for use in performance measures [1, 17] to create the *Attribute Grid* referenced in Stage 2 of the roadmap. Table 8.4 illustrates how specific characteristics of a PROM are used to evaluate its suitability for use in a PRO-PM [4].

Testing

While the test-driven tasks embedded in Stage 2 and Stage 3 of the PRO-PM roadmap have the shared purpose of promoting measure quality, they vary in focus and responsibility. Stage 2 tasks call for the measure developer to "ensure that sufficient testing (of the PROM) has occurred" [4], whereas Stage 3 focuses on testing the PRO-PM that *uses* the validated PROM. These tasks are distinctly different and essential to PRO-PM endorsement by CMS.

Table 8.4: Attribute grid for PROM comparison.

Attribute	PROM 1	PROM 2
Covers desired PROs reported from patient and/or caregiver perspective		
Outcome measured in PROM is the result of care for which relevant clinical quality is being measured		
Interpretable scores, defined and actionable cut points or targets, and anchors and/or defined meaningful change	*All relevant attributes of any number of candidate PROMs are compared by PRO-PM measure developers.*	
Clear conceptual and measurement models suitable for trending		
Psychometric Soundness: Reliability		
Psychometric Soundness: Validity		
Psychometric Soundness: Responsiveness		
Usability/Feasibility of Use: Low burden (e.g., length, time/effort to complete) and feasibility		
Usability/Feasibility of Use: Fits with standard of care and related workflows		
Usability/Feasibility of Use: ■ Cultural appropriateness ■ Language ■ Translated with culturally appropriate items		
Usability/Feasibility of Use: Availability of standardized clinical terminology and codes		
Usability/Feasibility of Use: Guidance on standardized data collection (including modes and methods)		

Source: Adapted from [4].

The PRO-PM roadmap demonstrates this distinction:

■ *Testing a PROM* occurs in Stage 2 and is the responsibility of the PROM developer.
■ *Testing a PRO-PM* occurs in Stage 3 and is the responsibility of the PRO-PM developer. Evaluation criteria include [4]:
  ■ Importance of the PRO-PM to the measurement goal defined in Stage 1
  ■ Scientific acceptability
  ■ Reliability of the PRO-PM
  ■ Validity of the PRO-PM (PROM validity, missing data, inadequate or absent case mix adjustment)

A distinction must be made when considering the reliability of PROMs versus the reliability of PRO-PMs. *Reliability of PROMs* refers to the repeatability and reproducibility of the actual questionnaire being used in the population of interest, usually obtained by repeat testing of an unchanged sample. *Reliability of the performance measure score* refers to the proportion of variation in the performance scores attributable to systematic differences across the measured entities in relation to random error ("signal-to-noise") [1]. Analysis of threats to PRO-PM validity and reliability must include consideration of case mix differences, risk adjustment, measure exclusions, and missing data or poor response rates [18].

Using PRO-PMs

Widespread adoption of PRO-PMs is contingent upon support and reinforcement at multiple levels across the healthcare industry. At the foundation, patients and their clinicians must understand the reporting value and have access to user-friendly technology to support consistent PROM collection and storage. Building upon this foundation:

- Health system accountability is implemented through *value-based regulatory programs* that reward the excellence of healthcare providers and incentivize improvement by associating quality metrics with upside and downside reimbursement adjustments.
- *Healthcare registries* support service providers with PROM data collection, analysis, and reporting for regulatory compliance. Ideally, a registry provides initial comparisons across member institutions of PRO-PM metrics to foster internal improvement activities, independent of regulatory reporting.
- *Healthcare system-level quality initiatives* promote PROM data collection for direct clinical use as well as quality improvement and regulatory reporting.

Regulatory Programs

Across the spectrum of CMS value-based quality initiatives, PRO-PMs are increasingly integrated at multiple levels. Providers, hospital inpatient facilities, outpatient facilities, and ambulatory surgery centers are incentivized to improve the quality of patient care while managing costs.

For Clinicians: The Merit-based Incentive Payment System   The Merit-based Incentive Payment System (MIPS) is a CMS Quality Payment Program that serves to adjust reimbursement payments to Medicare providers [19]. When PRO-PMs are added to the MIPS program, providers can offset the expense of PROM data collection through increased CMS reimbursement.

In 2023, CMS introduced MIPS Value Pathways (MVPs) as a new reporting option designed to simplify and streamline reporting to increase participation [20]. Of the initial twelve MVPs released, six included at least one PRO-PM in the set of quality measures available for reporting. Providers could also report improvement activities related to PROM data collection (e.g., Improvement Activity "Promote use of Patient-Reported Outcome Tools") [20].

For Hospitals and Outpatient Facilities: Quality Reporting Initiatives   CMS' hospital quality initiatives encompass organizations within the healthcare system and are designed to promote quality healthcare through accountability and public disclosure [21]. As PRO-PMs are added by CMS to quality initiatives, the patient perspective will increasingly be included in reimbursement adjustments and public reporting of quality metrics.

Adoption by CMS of the hospital-level risk-adjusted total hip arthroplasty/total knee arthroplasty PRO-PM (THA/TKA PRO-PM) for use in hospital Inpatient Quality Reporting (IQR) in 2023 marked the first-ever PRO-PM use in that program [22]. Adoption of a similar measure in Outpatient Quality Reporting (OQR) and Ambulatory Surgery Center Quality Reporting (ASCQR) programs [23] emphasizes the importance of strict adherence to a standardized process for PRO-PM development utilizing PROMs that are optimized for the intended use of the quality measure. The target population for this measure is large, and the statute requires PROM collection for each patient at two time points to allow assessment of change, or improvement, in health outcomes as measured by PROMs. The adoption of the THA/TKA PRO-PM in multiple quality reporting programs across an extended timeline for the large target population will result in large banks of valuable PROM data intended for use in quality improvement analytics. Late changes to a rigid PRO-PM structure, once data collection has started, can result in data fragmentation and reduced data quality.

Clinical Registries

A clinical registry is "an organized system for the collection, storage, retrieval, analysis, and dissemination of information on individual persons who have either a particular disease, a condition ... that predisposes to the occurrence of a health-related event, or prior exposure to substances ... known or suspected to cause adverse health effects" [24]. Compiled registry data serve many purposes, such as increasing safety and improving outcomes for patients while enforcing best practices for clinicians [25]. As registries integrate PROMs, they can compare quality across member institutions using PRO-PMs.

AAOS Registry Program   A good example of patient-reported outcome (PRO) data collection in registries is the American Association of Orthopedic Surgeons (AAOS) Registry Program, launched in 2017 with the mission "to improve orthopedic care through the collection, analysis, and reporting of actionable data" [25]. This program includes four AAOS registries and one shared registry, all with well-established PRO data collection programs. Across the five AAOS registries, participating surgeons and practices can submit data utilizing an AAOS Registry Program Authorized Vendor [26] and have access to national benchmarks, personalized dashboards, and advanced analytics [25]. A 2024 snapshot view of measures for each registry is summarized in Table 8.5. Note that PROMIS measures are well represented across

Table 8.5: PROM data collection in AAOS registries [25].

American Spine Registry [27]	Shoulder and Elbow Registry [28]	Fracture & Trauma Registry [29]	American Joint Replacement Registry [30]	AAOS Musculoskeletal Tumor Registry [31]
RECOMMENDED	**RECOMMENDED**	**RECOMMENDED**	**RECOMMENDED**	**RECOMMENDED**
PROMIS Global Health	PROMIS Global Health	PROMIS Global Health	PROMIS Global Health	PROMIS Global Health
VR-12	VR-12	VR-12	VR-12	VR-12
Numeric Rating Scale	ASES	PROMIS Physical Function	HOOS, JR.	MSTS
PROMIS Physical Function	SANE	Anatomic-specific PROMs for each module	KOOS, JR.	TESS
Oswestry Disability Index				
Neck Disability Index				
ACCEPTED	**ACCEPTED**	**ACCEPTED**	**ACCEPTED**	
PROMIS-29	PROMIS Upper Extremity	PROMIS-29	SF-36	
PROMIS Depression	PROMIS-29	PROMIS Anxiety	HOOS/KOOS	
PROMIS Anxiety	PROMIS Anxiety	PROMIS Depression	Oxford Hip and Knee Scores	
PROMIS Pain Interference	PROMIS Depression	PROMIS Pain Interference	Knee Society Knee Scoring System	
EQ-5D	PROMIS Pain Interference		Harris Hip Score	
			WOMAC	
			SF-12	
			EQ-5D	
			PROMIS-29	
			PROMIS Anxiety	
			PROMIS Depression	
			PROMIS Pain Interference	

Note: The lists of measures presented in Table 8.5 is based on information from the AAOS Registry Program website accessed on 28 December 2023.
Source: Adapted from Ref. [25].

the registries. Details about each of the PROMIS measures can be found on the HealthMeasures website.

Michigan Arthroplasty Registry Collaborative Quality Initiative (MARCQI)   MARCQI is a statewide specialty registry whose membership of 84 institutions represents more than 90% of the total joint replacement (TJR) procedures performed within the state of Michigan. MARCQI is dedicated to improving the quality of care for patients undergoing hip and knee replacement procedures in Michigan and manages a statewide consortium for the collaboration and sharing of best practices. By collecting and analyzing data, and then reporting results back to the providers, quality improvement initiatives are supported [32].

MARCQI works with providers across the state to collect PROM data. Michigan arthroplasty registry collaborative quality initiative (MARCQI) collects PROMIS Global Health, HOOS, JR (Hip dysfunction and Osteoarthritis Outcome Score for Joint Replacement) and KOOS, JR (Knee injury and Osteoarthritis Outcome Score for Joint Replacement) data, and several supplemental risk adjustment questions recommended by CMS. After collection, MARCQI provides physician and hospital "report cards" that include risk-adjusted comparisons of pre–post-PROM change. Early reports identified significant variation in PROM change across settings, and the collaboration will foster best practice discussions to support uniformly excellent outcomes. While MARCQI is a leader in the United States in including PROMs in comprehensive quality reports, internationally, PROMs have been collected and compared in quality reports for over a decade.

Qualified Clinical Data Registries   A Qualified Clinical Data Registry (QCDR) is a CMS-approved vendor that supports improving healthcare quality for their clients, in part through data collection and reporting to CMS for purposes of MIPS [33].

Approved QCDR vendors may also develop and submit new QCDR measures through a specialized CMS approval process. The benefit to clinicians is that many QCDR measures are specialty-based and may be more tailored to participant needs. CMS encourages QCDRs to harmonize similar measures, facilitating comparison and benchmarking [33].

Healthcare System Quality Improvement Programs

There is increasing interest in system-wide PROM data collection for use in routine patient care as well as in quality improvement programs, but adoption remains relatively low. Best practices in PROM implementation strategies used successfully by hundreds of orthopedic practices have been synthesized to provide specific guidance to other providers through each step in the implementation process [34]. Qualitative insights gained from PROM success stories in leading healthcare systems may help to overcome remaining barriers [35].

One example is the PROM program at Henry Ford Cancer, a tertiary cancer care center within the Henry Ford Health System. This program was launched in September 2019 with the establishment of a multi-specialty PRO committee. Domain-specific PROMIS measures (pain interference, fatigue, physical function, and depression) were selected to allow consistent use across all cancer types. With leadership support, physician champions, extensive training, and phased implementation, 23 of 38 clinical units were implemented between September 16, 2020, and July 23, 2021, with PROM data collected from 1666 patients over 2392 encounters [36].

Challenges and Opportunities

While patient-centered initiatives are widely recognized by healthcare leaders as a high priority, CMS-endorsed PRO-PMs remain under-actualized across performance measures and use in regulatory programs is limited [4].

Future efforts to drive widespread adoption of PRO-PMs in quality measurement will require continued collaboration in a multi-disciplinary approach to address:

- Technology challenges including interoperability and data sharing
- The role of technological advances in PRO-PM adoption
- PROM standardization
- Challenges of case mix/risk adjustment and health equity.

Interoperability and Data Standardization

Prerequisite to the widespread adoption of PRO-PMs for quality measurement is the availability of technology to support PROM capture, storage, interoperability, and data sharing, enabling benchmarking and comparison of PROM results across organizations.

The Office of the National Coordinator (ONC) for Health Information Technology partnered with the Agency for Healthcare Research and Quality (AHRQ) to create resources facilitating the availability of high-quality PROM data that are interoperable across organizations and facilities. Their work culminated in the 2020 publication of the *PRO Fast Healthcare Interoperability Resources Implementation Guide (PRO FHIR IG)*, a standardized specification for the collection, exchange, and integration of PRO data in electronic health record (EHR) systems. The guide includes an overview of the PRO Measure Lifecycle with the description of interactions for *adaptive* versus *fixed* measures and stepwise instructions on how to use FHIR to collect and store data in the EHR [5].

While technology requirements are described with guidance provided by the PRO FHIR IG, challenges remain. Early pilot testing performed during the development of the guide revealed issues that prevented successful implementation in a production environment. Recommended next steps covered in the 2020 report included further refinement of the PRO FHIR standard standardization of PROMs and increased use of Application Programming Interfaces (APIs) [37].

Ongoing progress can be seen in the custom integration of PROMIS CATs in the Epic EHR, which provides Epic users with seamless access to hundreds of PROMIS measures. This application is the result of collaboration between the PROMIS team and Epic and is natively integrated into Epic. The Epic PROMIS CAT application is built-in and includes automatic scoring using the ideal, precise response pattern scoring approach with score interpretation. As of 2024, a significant number of healthcare organizations were actively using the Epic PROMIS CAT application, with many academic medical centers participating in the Epic PROMIS Collaborative to share implementation experiences and develop best practices. Similar integration efforts with other EHR vendors are anticipated.

The Role of Technological Advances in PRO-PM Adoption

Current challenges unique to PRO-PM implementation that may be addressed through technology advances include [38]:

- PROM data collection can be disruptive to busy office staff and clinicians. Patient-centered technologies allow patients to complete PROMs from home using smartphones or other web-enabled devices to be stored in the EHR.
- Comparative PRO data availability to clinicians in real time at the point of care. When PROMs are available at the time of the office encounter, clinicians can review the data and discuss the health implications with patients. PROM use in care reinforces the value of PROM reporting to patients.
- PROMs reported between office visits that indicate the need for rapid attention, such as declining mobility or increasing pain, can trigger automated clinician alerts to evaluate patients and minimize morbidity.
- Enhanced PROM reporting can integrate advanced analytics and data visualization for meaningful communication and intuitive interpretation for both clinicians and patients.

PROM use in clinical care represents a paradigm shift for both patients and clinicians. Education on the optimal interpretation and use of PROMs is critical to assure that the data support communication and treatment decisions. For example, the physician's response of "Your survey results are back. Your score is 53." is not a clear answer to the patient who wonders: "Am I better?". Technology solutions to these challenges may range from creative color-coded reports through powerful artificial intelligence (AI) advances to collect patient-centered responses.

Future Applications of New Technology

Access to desktop, tablet, and mobile phone Americans with Disabilities Act (ADA)–compliant graphical interface tools can generate succinct, integrated dashboards to summarize information. However, patient numeracy varies widely, so alternate report strategies are needed. Advances in digital assistants such as Alexa, Siri, and Google Assistant have set the stage for a next-generation platform of friendly conversational patient education. Digital assistants grounded in shared terminology may be one approach to translating PROM scores into meaningful language.

While the current use of AI and machine learning (ML) tools is limited by the inconsistent availability of PROMs in large datasets, AI/ML applications may soon streamline communication and achieve widespread adoption and understanding of PRO-PMs. For example, AI technology provides opportunities for continuing research into more advanced IRT algorithms and even non-IRT CAT solutions that may further reduce patient burden and increase scoring precision and rapidity [39]. Traditional data collection modes may also progress using AI technology as an exercise directly between the patient and an EHR technology digital agent [40]. As an accelerator to health equity, any PRO implementation should also consider technology innovation to address language and health literacy challenges as future AI-powered translation tasks, which progress beyond current use as a simple mechanical process [41].

Standardizing PRO-PM Use in Quality Measurement

As PRO-PMs are utilized across diverse patient populations and treatment settings, new challenges emerge. For systems, integration of unique PROMs and assessment schedules becomes increasingly burdensome. For patients, completing multiple PROMs targeting specific treatments or conditions can also be increasingly burdensome. This is amplified when the PROM is not used to inform the patient's care and results (e.g., scores) are not shared back with the patient. There are multiple approaches for standardizing the PROMs used in PRO-PMs.

Disease-Agnostic PROMs

Many constructs assessed by PROMs (e.g., anxiety, fatigue, pain, physical function) are relevant in multiple patient populations and settings. When PRO-PMs use disease-agnostic PROMs, it creates opportunities for a patient to complete a PROM once and have it used in multiple ways. Furthermore, it creates a dataset within the EHR of how a given patient's symptom or function changes over time. This information can be utilized by different providers as well as made available to the patient for self-monitoring and increasing engagement in their care. PROMIS offers a library of disease-agnostic PROMs that can be used across age groups and patient populations [3].

Using a Common Metric

Another opportunity for standardizing PROMs is to focus on standardizing the *metric*, not the measure. Resources like the PRO Rosetta Stone (www.prosettastone.org) offer tables that enable translating the score from one PROM to the PROMIS metric. For example, a patient health questionnaire (PHQ-9) score, which is used to assess depression, can be translated into a PROMIS depression score. This has the potential for enabling multiple PROMs to be used in the same PRO-PM. Additional research is needed to identify best practices for using this approach.

Shared Measure Sets

A third approach to standardization is to create via consensus sets of measures to be used with specific patient populations. The International Consortium for Health Outcomes Measurement (ICHOM) assembles international teams of patients, clinicians, and researchers to select sets of PROMs measuring constructs that are meaningful to patients living with specific diseases or conditions. When organizations implement ICHOM sets of measures, it facilitates comparisons across patients and organizations internationally. The use of PROMs that are part of ICHOM sets in the construction of new PRO-PMs further facilitates comparisons and reduces the burden of implementation.

Case Mix/Risk Adjustment Challenges

Performance measures can be used *within* a single entity to monitor outcomes and to inform internal improvement efforts. In this case, a measure developer or policy maker may elect to case mix adjustment over time to compare PRO-PMs with a standardized patient mix to isolate the impact of the care provided from any change in patient demographic or clinical risks.

In contrast, policymakers use PRO-PMs to compare outcomes *across* health systems. In this situation, case mix and risk adjustment models are critical to assure evaluations compare the outcomes among comparable patient populations so that any outcome variation, positive or negative, can be attributed to the quality of care provided. For example, CMS and state-level adverse event analyses use case mix standardization or adjust for system-level (e.g., referral center, volume) and patient-level factors (e.g., age, sex, medical comorbidities) that are known to be associated with outcomes. For PRO-PMs, methodologists have documented that in addition to these socio-demographic and clinical factors, PROM scores *before* intervention are often associated with the PROM outcomes after intervention and may be included in statistical adjustments. For example, patients electing TJR surgery who are morbidly obese, have diabetes, and have lower pre-operative physical function scores are more likely to have poorer post-surgical PROM scores. Risk adjustment models may include these factors, and others, prior to comparing PRO-PMs across institutions. In addition, the proposed CMS rule for the introduction of PRO-PMs for TJR reimbursement includes comorbidities that are not available in the administrative international classification of diseases (ICD-10) codes such as co-occurring low back pain and pain in non-operative knees and hips. CMS specifies that post-TJR PROMs are collected approximately 12 months after the surgical procedure and that data are reported on 50% or more of patients at each site. Last, attention to equitable access and use of PROM reporting is critical to assuring representative patients are included in quality assessments.

In the future, CMS will provide reports on PRO-PMs for TJR surgeries performed in inpatient and outpatient settings.

Conclusion

The importance of patient-centered performance measurement has been recognized across the healthcare industry by regulatory agencies, payers, clinicians, and other healthcare leaders. Significant resources are in place to support the wide-scale development of PRO-PMs. Multi-year federally funded projects have produced detailed technical guidance, and technology advancements can be leveraged to address some of the remaining challenges. PROMIS and IRT-based linking of correlated measures into common metrics present an opportunity to accelerate the PRO-PM mission by providing standardized symptom and function scores across several clinical areas and enabling more assessment choices to healthcare organizations. A "tipping point" may soon be reached where the adoption of mandated PRO-PMs in regulatory initiatives in concert with the dedicated collaboration of clinicians and other healthcare leaders ensures that the voice of the patient is elevated and entrenched in quality measurement.

Discussion Questions

8.1 How can PROMs and PRO-PMs enhance healthcare quality measurement by incorporating the patient's voice, and what are the potential challenges in ensuring these metrics accurately reflect diverse patient priorities?

8.2 With the increasing adoption of electronic systems and IRT-based tools like PROMIS, how can PROMs be seamlessly integrated into clinical workflows without overburdening staff or patients?

8.3 Given the continued variability in PROMs, how can standardization initiatives like the PRO Rosetta Stone or ICHOM sets improve consistency in quality measurement?

8.4 What are the ethical and methodological considerations when developing risk adjustment models for PRO-PMs, particularly in ensuring fair comparisons across institutions and populations with different baseline health conditions?

8.5 How can emerging technologies, such as AI and digital assistants, be leveraged to improve patient engagement, enhance data collection processes, and overcome barriers to broader adoption of PRO-PMs in regulatory programs?

Acknowledgements

This work was supported in part by the Northwestern University Outcomes Measurement and Survey Core and a Cancer Center Support Grant (NCI CA060553).

References

1 Cella, D., Hahn, E.A., Jensen, S.E. et al. (2015). *Patient-Reported Outcomes in Performance Measurement*. Research Triangle Park, NC: RTI Press.

2 Centers for Medicare & Medicaid Services (CMS). Supplemental material to CMS MMS hub: patient-reported outcome measures. https://mmshub.cms.gov/sites/default/files/Patient-Reported-Outcome-Measures.pdf (accessed 28 December 2023).

3 HealthMeasures Intro to PROMIS. https://www.healthmeasures.net/explore-measurement-systems/promis (accessed 1 January 2024).

4 National Quality Forum (2022). Building a roadmap from patient-reported outcome measures to patient-reported outcome performance measures: technical guidance-updated final draft. https://www.qualityforum.org/Projects/n-r/PRO-PM/Final_Technical_Guidance_Report_11302022.aspx (accessed 26 April 2025 2023).

5 HL7 (2019). FHIR implementation guide (Release 0.2.0): patient reported outcomes FHIR implementation guide. https://hl7.org/fhir/us/patient-reported-outcomes/2019May/ (accessed 28 December 2023).

6 Centers for Medicare & Medicaid Services (CMS). Supplemental material to CMS MMS hub: risk adjustment and risk stratification in quality measurement. https://mmshub.cms.gov/sites/default/files/Risk-Adjustment-in-Quality-Measurement.pdf (accessed 19 December 2024).

7 Centers for Medicare & Medicaid Services Glossary. https://www.cms.gov/glossary (accessed 19 December 2024).

8 Bech, P. (1993). Quality of life measurements in chronic disorders. *Psychother. Psychosom.* 59 (1): 1–10.

9 Cella, D.F., Tulsky, D.S., Gray, G. et al. (1993). The Functional Assessment of Cancer Therapy scale: development and validation of the general measure. *J. Clin. Oncol.* 11 (3): 570–579.

10 Cohen, M.E. and Marino, R.J. (2000). The tools of disability outcomes research functional status measures. *Arch. Phys. Med. Rehabil.* 81 (12 Suppl 2): S21–S29.

11 Gapstur, R.L. (2007). Symptom burden: a concept analysis and implications for oncology nurses. *Oncol. Nurs. Forum* 34 (3): 673–680. https://doi.org/10.1188/07.ONF.673-680.

12 Short, S.E. and Mollborn, S. (2015). Social determinants and health behaviors: conceptual frames and empirical advances. *Curr. Opin. Psychol.* 5: 78–84. https://doi.org/10.1016/j.copsyc.2015.05.002.

13 Fayers, P. and Machin, D. (2007). *Quality of Life: The Assessment, Analysis and Interpretation of Patient-reported Outcomes*, 2e. Chichester: Wiley.

14 HealthMeasures Measurement science: computer adaptive tests (CATs). https://www.healthmeasures.net/resource-center/measurement-science/computer-adaptive-tests-cats/ (accessed 19 December 2024).

15 Papuga, M.O., Dasilva, C., McIntyre, A. et al. (2017). Large-scale clinical implementation of PROMIS computer adaptive testing with direct incorporation into the electronic medical record. *Health. Syst. (Basingstoke).* 7 (1): 1–12. https://doi.org/10.1057/s41306-016-0016-1.

16 Centers for Medicare & Medicaid Services (2023). Blueprint for the CMS measures management system. https://mmshub.cms.gov/blueprint-measure-lifecycle-overview (accessed 28 December 2023).

17 Cella, D., Hahn, E.A., Jensen, S.E. et al. (2012). Methodological issues in the selection, administration and use of patient-reported outcomes in performance measurement in health care settings. National Quality Forum 2012.

18 Deutsch, A., Smith, L., Gage, B. et al. (2012). *Patient-Reported Outcomes in Performance Measurement.* Prepared by RTI International and Brookings Institution. Washington, DC: NQF. Available at https://www.qualityforum.org/Publications/2012/12/Patient-Reported_Outcomes_Final_Report.aspx.

19 Centers for Medicare & Medicaid Services (CMS). MIPS explore measures – QPP. Quality payment program. https://qpp.cms.gov/mips/explore-measures?tab=qualityMeasures&py=2022 (accessed 29 December 2023).

20 Centers for Medicare & Medicaid Services (CMS). Quality payment program. Explore MIPS value pathways (MVPs). https://qpp.cms.gov/mips/explore-mips-value-pathways (accessed 28 December 2023).

21 Centers for Medicare & Medicaid Services (CMS). Hospital quality initiative. Quality initiatives – general information. https://www.cms.gov/medicare/quality/initiatives (accessed 19 December 2024).

22 Centers for Medicare and Medicaid Services (CMS). QualityNet hospitals-inpatient measures: THA/TKA PRO-PM overview. https://qualitynet.cms.gov/inpatient/measures/THA_TKA (accessed 19 December 2024).

23 Federal Register 88 FR 81540 (2023). Medicare program: hospital outpatient prospective payment and ambulatory surgical center payment systems (Rule). https://www.federalregister.gov/documents/2023/11/22/2023-24293/medicare-program-hospital-outpatient-prospective-payment-and-ambulatory-surgical-center-payment (accessed 19 December 2024).

24 American Academy of Orthopaedic Surgeons. AAOS registry program frequently asked questions. https://www.aaos.org/registries/program-details/faqs/ (accessed 19 December 2024).

25 American Academy of Orthopaedic Surgeons (AAOS). About the AAOS registry program. https://www.aaos.org/registries/registry-program/about-the-aaos-registry-program (accessed 19 December 2024).

26 American Academy of Orthopaedic Surgeons. AAOS registry program authorized vendors. https://www.aaos.org/registries/program-details/authorized-vendor-program (accessed 19 December 2024).

27 American Spine Registry. About the American Spine Registry. https://www.americanspineregistry.org/about-the-american-spine-registry/about-us/ (accessed 19 December 2024).

28 American Academy of Orthopaedic Surgeons. The AAOS shoulder & elbow registry: improving orthopaedic care through data. https://www.aaos.org/registries/registry-program/fracture-and-trauma-registry/ (accessed 19 December 2024).

29 American Academy of Orthopaedic Surgeons. The AAOS fracture & trauma registry: improving orthopaedic care through data. https://www.aaos.org/registries/registry-program/fracture-and-trauma-registry/ (accessed 19 December 2024).

30 American Academy of Orthopaedic Surgeons. The AAOS American Joint Replacement Registry: improving orthopaedic care through data. https://www.aaos.org/registries/registry-program/american-joint-replacement-registry/ (accessed 19 December 2024).

31 American Academy of Orthopaedic Surgeons. The AAOS musculoskeletal tumor registry: improving orthopaedic care through data. https://www.aaos.org/registries/registry-program/musculoskeletal-tumor-registry/ (accessed 19 December 2024).

32 Michigan Arthroplasty Registry Collaborative Quality Initiative. https://marcqi.org/ (accessed 18 December 2023).

33 Centers for Medicare and Medicaid Services (CMS) (2018). Measures management system: a brief overview of qualified clinical data registries. Measurement management system newsletter-508. https://www.cms.gov/Medicare/Quality-Initiatives-Patient-Assessment-instruments/MMS/Downloads/A-Brief-Overview-of-Qualified-Clinical-Data-Registries.pdf (accessed 19 December 2024).

34 Franklin, P.D., Bond, C.P., Rothrock, N.E., and Cella, D. (2021). Strategies for effective implementation of patient-reported outcome measures in arthroplasty practice. *J. Bone Joint Surg. Am.* 103 (24): e97. https://doi.org/10.2106/JBJS.20.02072.

35 Hyland, C.J., Guo, R., Dhawan, R. et al. (2022). Implementing patient-reported outcomes in routine clinical care for diverse and underrepresented patients in the United States. *J. Patient Rep. Outcomes* 6: 20. https://doi.org/10.1186/s41687-022-00428-z.

36 Tam, S., Zatirka, T., Neslund-Dudas, C. et al. (2023). Real time patient-reported outcome measures in patients with cancer: early experience within an integrated health system. *Cancer Med.* 12 (7): 8860–8870. https://doi.org/10.1002/cam4.5635.

37 The Office of the National Coordinator for Health Information Technology (2020). Advancing the collection and use of patient-reported outcomes through Health Information Technology: final report. Prepared by ESAC, Inc. for the Office of the National Coordinator for Health Information Technology under Contract No. HHSP233201500103I HHSP23337002T.

38 Jensen, R.E., Rothrock, N.E., DeWitt, E.M. et al. (2015). The role of technical advances in the adoption and integration of patient-reported outcomes in clinical care. *Med. Care* 53 (2): 153–159. https://doi.org/10.1097/MLR.0000000000000289.

39 Mujtaba, D. and Mahapatra, N. (2020). Artificial intelligence in computerized adaptive testing. *2020 International Conference on Computational Science and Computational Intelligence (CSCI)*, Las Vegas, NV, USA, pp. 649–654. doi: 10.1109/CSCI51800.2020.00116; keywords: {deep learning;cats;scientific computing;reinforcement learning;organizations;natural language processing;inference algorithms} url: https://doi.ieeecomputersociety.org/10.1109/CSCI51800.2020.00116.

40 Tan, Z., He, Q., and Feng, S. (2023). The collision of ChatGPT and traditional medicine: a perspective from bibliometric analysis. *Int. J. Surg.* 109 (11): 3713–3714. Published 1 November 2023. https://doi.org/10.1097/JS9.0000000000000662.

41 Bakdash, L., Abid, A., Gourisankar, A. et al. (2023). Chatting beyond ChatGPT: advancing equity through AI-driven language interpretation. *J. Gen. Intern. Med.* 39. https://doi.org/10.1007/s11606-023-08497-6.

9

Measuring Equity in Health and Healthcare

Jill A. Marsteller [1,2,3], Christina A. Vincent [2], Andrew Anderson [1], John Jackson [2,4], J. Matthew Austin [3,5], and Lisa A. Cooper [2,6,7]

[1] Department of Health Policy and Management, Johns Hopkins Bloomberg School of Public Health, Baltimore, MD, USA

[2] Department of Medicine, Johns Hopkins Center for Health Equity, Johns Hopkins School of Medicine, Baltimore, MD, USA

[3] Armstrong Institute for Patient Safety and Quality, Johns Hopkins School of Medicine, Baltimore, MD, USA

[4] Departments of Epidemiology, Mental Health, and Biostatistics, Johns Hopkins Bloomberg School of Public Health, Baltimore, MD, USA

[5] Department of Anesthesiology and Critical Care Medicine, Johns Hopkins School of Medicine, Baltimore, MD, USA

[6] Department of Health, Behavior and Society, Johns Hopkins Bloomberg School of Public Health, Baltimore, MD, USA

[7] Johns Hopkins School of Nursing, Baltimore, MD, USA

Introduction

Issues of health and healthcare equity have reached a critical juncture. While more people became aware of and concerned about structural and cultural racism in recent years, antithetical forces have begun to push back on the need for attention to historic inequities that have led to disparities in health and healthcare. One area where advances have been made, and can be a lasting improvement, is in the appropriate measurement of disparities in healthcare delivery. Penman-Aguilar and colleagues (2016) echoed Frieden (2013), "What is not measured cannot readily be remedied; thus, the provision of accurate and useful data is foundational" [1, 2] (p. S34). This chapter provides an overview of the state of healthcare equity in the United States and then provides a review of the current state of equity measurement in healthcare, including measurement of constructs of race, ethnicity, social determinants of health, and gaps among groups. We conclude with a discussion of recommendations for healthcare equity measurement.

Based on Braveman (2014), health equity is a state where healthcare achieves "the highest possible standard of health for all people and giving special attention to the needs of those at greatest risk of poor health, based on social conditions" [3]. Although we aspire to the highest standard, implicit in equity is the need to identify and dismantle unjust differences. Thus, a critical understanding in measuring health equity is what constitutes a disparity. It is a difference wherein social groups that have endured long-standing social, political, and economic disadvantages are at further disadvantage with respect to the outcome (e.g., health status or healthcare utilization) [3]. The National Institute of Minority Health and Health Disparities (NIMHD) explicitly emphasizes socially disadvantaged groups as disparity populations, which include racial and ethnic minoritized groups, underserved rural residents, persons with lower socioeconomic status, and sexual and gender minorities [4]. A disparity reflects a "concern for social justice" [3]. Thus, not every difference among groups is a disparity. We note, however, that while the most socially advantaged group is often used as a reference group in assessing disparity, some use the healthiest group, which may better reflect attainable outcomes [3]. The notion of equitable care quality spans across domains of access to, use of, and treatment within the healthcare system. To achieve health equity, we must pursue equitable healthcare. This ultimately focuses on giving to each as they need, so that equitable outcomes of care can be realized.

Fundamentally, the highest care quality is not reached if some patients receive substandard care. The concept of sameness in quality, however, is by itself insufficient if the level of quality has not reached the "highest possible standard" or if the outcomes of healthcare are still disparate because "special attention" was not given to those at greatest risk. Healthcare has long observed boundaries of clinic or hospital walls but today has accepted the possibility and importance of reaching into the community to help patients combat negative social determinants of health [5, 6].

This notion of achieving health equity raises an important question: What would health equity look like if we had it? The Institute of Medicine (IOM), now known as the National Academy of Medicine (NAM), detailed six aims for the healthcare system in *Crossing the Quality Chasm* [7] and, in doing so, established a persistent caliber to which all health services should be held. Health services should be (1) safe, (2) effective, (3) patient-centered, (4) timely, (5) efficient, and (6) equitable [8]. By defining these six domains, health services researchers set core domains in which to create measures that assess care. Two years later, in 2003, the IOM published a landmark report, *Unequal Treatment: Confronting Racial and Ethnic Disparities in Health Care* [9]. This detailed systemic racial and ethnic disparities in all aspects of American healthcare, calling attention to the history of worsening health outcomes for marginalized groups [8]. By defining equitable care and explicitly presenting areas of focus, the IOM initiated a practice that others would soon follow. The incorporation of equity into meaningful measurement, however, has proven complex to achieve. Throughout this chapter, we explore current measures in health equity and the key aspects to creating successful measures in the future.

Current State of Affairs: Long-Standing Inequities by Many Measures

Twenty years have passed since the release of *Unequal Treatment*. While there has been headway, the Agency for Healthcare Research and Quality (AHRQ's) annual Healthcare Quality and Disparities Report [10] states that disparities in outcomes for marginalized groups still remain. Additional evidence documenting these disparities can be found in the National Academies report *Ending Unequal Treatment*, released in 2024 – an analysis that details the progress made since *Unequal Treatment* was released in 2003 and opportunities to shrink the existing gap in health outcomes and care [11]. Included in this are recommendations of policies and programs that work toward long-lasting, sustainable solutions including improved data sharing and investments to build the evidence base of health equity research, funding for effective healthcare delivery programs, and establishing accountability systems to ensure equitable care services [11]. The Urban Institute also released an analysis of race and ethnicity data, which comments on the crucial role data play in the solution to achieving equity in healthcare [12]. Of the many barriers mentioned, James et al. (2023) identified gaps in action that lead to gaps in demographic data – lack of engagement with communities, lack of data sharing and interoperability, and lack of consistency in public reporting [12]. Along with this, there is little information collected on the demographics of clinicians and other health professionals, which research shows is relevant to physician–patient relationships [13–15]. Solutions were proposed to improve data collection and integrity. For improved data collection, researchers suggested providing optional, respectfully worded questions about race and ethnicity in surveys to obtain authentic results and primarily focusing efforts on the most disparate health outcomes. Additionally, Urban Institute researchers stressed the importance of collecting clinician race and ethnicity data and making these data available to patients if desired, citing the role of race concordance in patient ratings of satisfaction, participatory decision-making in care, and patient preferences [11, 12, 16, 17]. They recommended that health systems, professional associations, and regulatory bodies with health plans or consumers work to address technical, regulatory, and privacy barriers to collecting these data.

In recent years, the NIMHD created a research framework to conceptualize the causal factors that perpetuate health disparities for marginalized populations (Table 9.1) [18]. It is important to concentrate on the levels of care we can quantify, that is, measure and analyze. This focuses attention on aspects such as quality of care and availability of services, as well as individual and interpersonal levels of influence within the biological, behavioral, and sociocultural domains. Each of the factors listed within the matrix is areas where we have current methods of measurement and, importantly, can measure change in these data over time. Some longitudinal datasets allow researchers to capture the entire equity picture by analyzing care and outcomes within subpopulations.

Measurement of Health and Healthcare Equity

Operational Definitions and Measure Development

The development of measures for assessing health equity has relied on operational definitions from diverse sources, including researchers, government bodies, and foundations, leading to a variation in definitions. Starting in the 1980s, awareness of inequities in health and healthcare began to garner national attention [19]. National reports such as the AHRQ's National Healthcare Quality and Disparities Report (NHQDR) [10] and Healthy People 2030 [20] point out key groups facing disparities and marginalization.

A measure is a simple number, while a metric specifies numbers that describe a relationship, such as blood pressure (BP) control rates (e.g., the number of people with a BP of 140/90 relative to all people with a diagnosis of hypertension). As is commonplace throughout health services research,

Table 9.1: National institute on minority health and health disparities research framework.

		Levels of influence			
		Individual	**Interpersonal**	**Community**	**Society**
Domains of influence	Biological	Biological vulnerability and mechanisms	Caregiver–child interactions, family microbiome	Community illness exposure, herd immunity	Sanitation, immunization, pathogen exposure
	Behavioral	Health behaviors and coping strategies	Family functioning, school/work functioning	Community functioning, policies, and laws	Policies and laws
	Physical environment	Personal environment	Household environment, school/work environment	Community environment, community resources	Society structure
	Sociocultural environment	Socioeconomics, limited English, cultural identity, response to discrimination	Social networks, family/peer norms, interpersonal discrimination	Community norms, local structural discrimination	Social norms, structural discrimination
	Healthcare system	Insurance coverage, health literacy, treatment preferences	Patient–clinician relationship, medicaldecision-making	Availability of services, safety net services	Quality of care, healthcare policies
Health outcomes		Individual health	Family/organizational health	Community health	Population health

Source: NIMHD Research Framework Details [18] / https://www.nimhd.nih.gov/about/overview/research-framework/nimhd-framework.html (accessed 28 January 2025) / US Department of Health & Human Services / Public Domain.

the words "metric" and "measure" can be used interchangeably. We use the term "indicator," or sociodemographic indicator, to describe the use of these measures/metrics as a gauge to monitor health status across factors such as race, ethnicity, and primary language, as defined by the National Committee for Quality Assurance (NCQA) [21].

As of 2024, literature around best practices for health equity measurement remains limited. The *status quo* methodology is to express the differences in health outcomes between populations and document the difference, comparing one group to another (often the white population to marginalized groups). For example, Healthy People 2030 pinpointed 23 leading health indicators summarizing the major causes of death and disease in the United States across the lifespan, including infant death, drug overdose deaths, possession of medical insurance, use of oral healthcare, consumption of calories from added sugars (e.g., in those over 2 years old), tobacco use (e.g., among adolescents), new diagnoses of diabetes, and hypertension control (e.g., among adults) [20]. By comparing such measures among populations, these data drive health equity researchers and system leaders to describe gaps and further study the causal factors, as well as give policymakers and legislators an avenue to focus attention and legislation.

Approaches that start from a definition of equity (such as the *Robert Wood Johnson Foundation's* goal to reduce and eventually eradicate disparities in health and their determinants) [22] still underscore the vital role of measuring disparities to gauge progress toward health equity. Conceptually, health equity resides on a theoretical plane, rendering it somewhat intangible and challenging to quantify directly. Therefore, in practice, health equity is often operationalized by comparing outcomes between historically marginalized groups and their counterparts who have traditionally not faced the same level of exclusion. This approach, however, oversimplifies the complex reality that individuals possess a myriad of attributes that can both positively and negatively affect their social status and, subsequently, their health outcomes. The nuanced interplay among these attributes is seldom captured by quantitative measures, indicating a gap in how disparities are comprehensively understood and addressed.

AHRQ delineates a disparity as the entirety of differences between groups assigned to various social categories, such as race or ethnicity, highlighting the challenges in adjusting for poor and problematic data [23]. The NAM, on the other hand, categorizes a disparity as all differences that are not attributable to health status or patient preferences (the latter are considered "allowable" factors; other factors related to injustice are "unallowable") [24]. Furthermore, some researchers advocate for a definition that encompasses any difference between individuals assigned to distinct social categories, after accounting for as many other health-influencing factors as possible, known as the residual direct effect [25]. This nuanced approach to defining disparities underscores the complexity of attributing differences in health outcomes to social injustices, emphasizing the need for theory-driven guidance to navigate the empirical and causal relationships inherent in this endeavor.

The evolution and refinement of health equity measures in healthcare organizations and systems have led to a proliferation of indicators. Indicators sourced from a range of data types such as administrative claims and survey responses aim to capture different facets of equity, including considerations of race, ethnicity, socioeconomic status, and disability. Measure developers make choices based on their operational definitions of a disparity and its context. This includes the selection of a baseline for disparity measurement, the choice to assess disparities in absolute or relative terms, a determination whether to focus on positive or negative health outcomes, the identification of an analytical approach (whether to examine disparities within individual groups, to compare groups directly, or to use a composite measure), and a decision about weighting groups within composite measures (or not). In the case of weighting, the literature describes the potential benefits of using this approach to incentivize equity by emphasizing the need to improve care for smaller or marginalized groups, while ensuring that this emphasis has no effect on the quality of care for other groups [26]. Each choice plays a crucial role in defining the magnitude and direction of the disparities measured, thus shaping the understanding and intervention strategies for health equity.

Measurement Approaches

In 2021, the Office of the Assistant Secretary for Planning and Evaluation (ASPE) at the US Department of Health & Human Services (HHS) published a comprehensive effort to identify and refine existing approaches for measuring health equity [27]. The project was motivated by the need to address disparities in healthcare quality and outcomes associated with social risk factors such as socioeconomic status, race, and ethnicity. The report details a literature review and expert panel input that identified ten health equity measurement approaches. Similarly, amid a landscape of existing measures, the NCQA identified several approaches that they felt demonstrated notable promise, including the health equity metric, the population health performance index, Humana's composite measure, and the health equity summary score.

We compiled current measurement approaches in Table 9.2. In addition, we interpret their fit into the NIMHD's Research Framework to conceptualize how each measure approaches health equity research. These different approaches have general aims in common to evaluate how well healthcare organizations meet standards that promote equitable care, assess disparities in care quality and outcomes, and summarize the extent to which care quality contributes to reducing health disparities at the population level.

Each approach is designed with specific criteria for evaluating health equity, including the evidence base, usability, measurement equivalence, breadth of applicability, reliability, and impact. The approaches vary in their focus, with some emphasizing structural measures within healthcare organizations and others focusing on patient experiences, clinical outcomes, and overall quality of care. New measures continue to emerge.

Guidance for Measure Development and Compliance

Through a detailed analysis of various methodologies employed within Medicare and Medicaid, the NCQA developed a structured approach for creating health equity measures, as outlined in their review of measurement and scoring methodologies [36]. This approach involves four crucial steps: (1) identification of social determinants of health indicators, (2) selection of a reference or comparison group, (3) choice of healthcare quality

Table 9.2: Current health equity measurement approaches.

Measurement approach	Description	NIMHD Levels/domains of influence	Examples of /metrics within measurement approach
Measurement framework for evaluating how well an organization meets national CLAS[a] standards (HHS[b] OMH[c]) [25, 28]	This approach assesses organizational adherence to standards promoting culturally and linguistically appropriate services	▪ Level of influence: sociocultural environment ▪ Domain of influence: interpersonal	▪ Clinician/group's cultural competence or health literacy practices based on the CAHPS[d] ▪ Percentage of patient visits and admissions in which preferred spoken language for healthcare is screened and recorded ▪ Clinician and staff perceptions of organizational commitment to cultural competency [29]
NQF[e] Disparities-Sensitive Measure Assessment [25, 30]	Identifies existing quality measures suitable for health equity comparisons	▪ Level of influence: individual ▪ Domain of influence: healthcare system	▪ Influenza immunization ▪ Cervical cancer screening ▪ Median time from emergency department arrival to electrocardiogram ▪ Hemoglobin A1c testing ▪ Controlled high blood pressure within the measurement year
AHRQ[f] National Healthcare Quality and Disparities Report [10, 25]	Provides annual reports on healthcare quality and disparities across various dimensions including race and ethnicity	▪ Domain of influence: healthcare system ▪ Levels of influence: all levels	▪ Adults with an appointment in the last 12 months who sometimes/never got an appointment as soon as needed ▪ Adult postoperative sepsis per 1,000 elective surgery admissions ▪ Adult hospital patients reporting poor communication about discharge ▪ Women <70 treated for breast cancer with breast-conserving surgery who received radiation within 1 year of diagnosis ▪ Live-born infants with low birth weight (less than 2,500 g) ▪ People without a usual source of care for financial or insurance reasons ▪ Virtual visits per 1,000 substance abuse visits to HRSA[g]-supported health centers

Table 9.2: (Continued)

Measurement approach	Description	NIMHD Levels/domains of influence	Examples of /metrics within measurement approach
CMS[h] OMH Mapping Medicare Disparities (MMD) Tool [25, 31]	A tool for visualizing disparities in health outcomes and conditions across geographic areas	▪ Level of influence: societal ▪ Domain of influence: healthcare system	▪ Prevalence rates and costs ▪ Hospitalization rates ▪ AHRQ prevention quality indicators (PQI) ▪ Readmission rates ▪ Mortality rates ▪ Emergency department visit rates ▪ AHRQ patient safety indicators (PSIs)
CMS OMH reporting of CAHPS and HEDIS[i] data stratified by race and ethnicity for Medicare beneficiaries [25, 32]	Offers insights into disparities in patient experiences and healthcare effectiveness through stratified reporting	▪ Levels of influence: individual and interpersonal ▪ Domain of influence: healthcare system	▪ Patient experience measures, such as getting care quickly and getting needed care ▪ Clinical care measures such as continuous beta-blocker treatment after a heart attack, rheumatoid arthritis measurement, and kidney disease monitorization
Minnesota healthcare disparities report: Eliminating health disparities initiative report to the legislature [25, 33]	An annual report detailing disparities in care quality among various populations within Minnesota	▪ Level of influence: individual ▪ Domain of influence: healthcare system	▪ Optimal diabetes care ▪ Optimal asthma control, in both adults and children ▪ Colorectal cancer screening ▪ Adult depression: follow-up, response, and remission at 6 and 12 months ▪ Adolescent mental health and/or depression screening
CMS assessment of hospital disparities for dual-eligible patients [25, 34]	Evaluates hospital performance in providing equitable care to patients eligible for both Medicare and Medicaid	▪ Level of influence: individual and interpersonal ▪ Domain of influence: healthcare system	▪ Breast and colorectal cancer screenings ▪ Medication adherence for cardiovascular disease ▪ Diabetes, blood sugar control ▪ Osteoporosis management in women who had a fracture ▪ Follow-up after a hospital stay for mental illness ▪ Medication reconciliation after inpatient admission ▪ Avoiding potentially harmful drug–disease interactions ▪ Older adults' access to preventative/ambulatory services

(Continued)

Table 9.2: (Continued)

Measurement approach	Description	NIMHD Levels/domains of influence	Examples of /metrics within measurement approach
CMS OMH health equity summary score (HESS) [25, 35]	A composite score reflecting the extent of equitable care provided across different measures and populations	▪ Domain of influence: healthcare system ▪ Levels of influence: individual and interpersonal	▪ MA and PDP[j] CAHPS measures such as getting appointments and care quickly and doctors who communicate well ▪ HEDIS measures such as cancer screenings and BMI assessment ▪ Diabetes: blood sugar controlled
HCAHPS[k] HESS [36]	Composite of two scores (cross-sectional and improvement scores) that measure performance on different aspects of patient experience (HCAHPS) for different groups of patients	▪ Level of influence: interpersonal ▪ Domain of influence: healthcare system	▪ Hospital characteristics such as number of beds, overall HCAPS rating, teaching, non- or for-profit ▪ Patient characteristics such as race and preferred primary language
Zimmerman's health-related quality of life approach to assessing health equity, health equity metric (HEM) [25, 37]	Focuses on assessing disparities in health-related quality of life outcomes	▪ Level of influence: societal ▪ Domain of influence: healthcare system	▪ "Healthy days" as derived from the CDC's[l] health-related quality of life scale, based off of data from the 2017 Behavioral Risk Factor Surveillance System data
Zimmerman and Anderson approach to evaluating trends over time in health equity [25, 38]	Analyzes trends in health equity over time across various measures	▪ Level of influence: interpersonal ▪ Domain of influence: sociocultural environment	▪ Black–white disparity ▪ Income disparity ▪ Health justice ▪ A health equity measure weighted by the total difference between the determined health of the individual and the best achievable health
Population health performance index [39, 40]	Conducts comparisons across state populations, focusing on two primary dimensions: health inequity and overall population health	▪ Level of influence: societal ▪ Domains of influence: sociocultural and healthcare system	▪ Health metrics: infant mortality ▪ Binarized dimension of social inequality: educational attainment, race, and ethnicity

Table 9.2: (Continued)

Measurement approach	Description	NIMHD Levels/domains of influence	Examples of /metrics within measurement approach
Humana's approach [35, 41]	A composite measure created from eight health behavior metrics across Medicare advantage plans	■ Level of influence: community ■ Domain of influence: individual	■ Medication adherence ■ Preventative care ■ Diabetes care ■ Vaccination status ■ Attending a primary care visit
Leapfrog [42]	A structural measure that assesses whether hospitals and ambulatory surgery centers are taking the steps necessary to understand potential inequities in their care delivery	■ Level of influence: all ■ Domain of influence: healthcare system	■ Facility training for staff on best practices for SDoH collection ■ Facility sharing of updates with BoD on equity progress

[a] CLAS: Culturally and Linguistically Appropriate Services
[b] HHS: US Department of Health and Human Services
[c] OMH: Office of Minority Health
[d] CAHPS: Consumer Assessment of Healthcare Providers and Systems
[e] NQF: National Quality Forum
[f] AHRQ: Agency for Healthcare Research and Quality
[g] HRSA: Health Resources and Services Administration
[h] CMS: Center for Medicare & Medicaid Services
[i] HEDIS: Healthcare Effectiveness Data and Information Set
[j] MA and PDP CAHPS: Medicare Advantage and Prescription Drug Plan Consumer Assessment of Healthcare Providers and Systems
[k] HCAHPS: Hospital Consumer Assessment of Healthcare Providers and Systems
[l] CDC: Center for Disease Control a. CLAS: Culturally and Linguistically Appropriate Services

metrics/measures, and (4) application of benchmarks to contextualize results against national averages [36].

The Leapfrog Group developed a health equity standard that measures a facility's compliance with six important steps for measuring and improving health equity. The steps include (1) collecting sociodemographic data from patients; (2) training staff on how to best collect sociodemographic data from patients; (3) stratifying quality measures using the patient self-reported demographic data; (4) identifying any disparities and starting to address any that are found; (5) regularly sharing updates on this work with the hospital's or ambulatory surgery center's Board of Directors; and (6) sharing efforts about this work on their public website [39].

Recommendations for Good Measures and Measurement in Health Equity

Developing Strong Measures and Metrics/Measures

At a minimum, for a measure to be meaningful, quality metrics/measures should have a well-defined denominator and a well-defined period of follow-up for assessing outcomes. The denominator is important for interpreting the target population to which the results apply. In practice (for example, in a quality improvement dashboard), clinicians who feel the denominator of patients assigned to them is inaccurate will not believe any quality metric calculated over that denominator. Also, the follow-up period is important for understanding whether the quality issues are immediate, short term, or long term, which has important implications for designing policies and interventions to improve equity in the quality of healthcare. At times, covariate adjustment (e.g., reflecting need for services) may be required and it is important to provide appropriate justifications, ideally guided by a conceptual model for how these covariates relate to quality-based outcomes. Below, we describe special considerations that accompany each of these factors.

One common challenge of measuring equity is the available sample size among different subgroups. Some healthcare organizations may have a small number of patients within a particular sociodemographic subgroup, which can make it difficult to understand, with statistical confidence, whether a noted difference in quality in that subpopulation is a true difference in quality or simply an appearance of difference. Two potential approaches for increasing sample size are to use longer time periods for measurement (e.g., using a five-year time period instead of a three-year time period) and/or to aggregate smaller subgroups together. Each approach improves the statistical power to detect differences, but has its own drawbacks, including masking any changes in performance over time and understanding differences among members of the aggregated subgroups.

Within this notion of sample sizes comes the idea that ideal health equity metrics/measures would include intersectional approaches (e.g., consideration of race and gender together, which acknowledges the fact that people have characteristics in combination and may be minoritized in one aspect of their identity but may represent a dominant group in another characteristic). In addition, appropriate reference groups should be situationally defined. In any score, a benchmark serves as a foundational tool for evaluation, one that should be included in the creation of new health equity measures. Within health systems (especially Medicare and Medicaid), setting performance goals is critical to the greater evaluation of quality of healthcare services and can provide insight into where gaps arise. Composite scores prove beneficial in their summarization of multiple single-measure values, distilling data points from a larger set and creating a value that is easier to interpret. However, when considering the simplicity of calculation – a crucial aspect of data validity and integrity – the utilization of these complex scoring methods proves less viable on a wider scale. While their output creates a maximum impact, the availability of these composite scores relies on all reporting units to obtain each individual value, which would necessitate the tools and resources required to record each individual data point. Unless the collection of all necessary data is required of each reporting unit, and funding is provided to ensure the software and capabilities to collect them, widespread utilization of composite scores may prove to be an unrealistic venture.

The importance of these composite scores and single-variable benchmarks is their ability to show change over time. If these composite scores become more widely incorporated into health equity practices, several years' experience would be required to present their longitudinal trend, which, as mentioned, proves difficult in smaller sample sizes where these outcomes are masked. However, generally this type of statistical presentation may be set best in smaller communities, rather than retrofitted to assess the national state of health disparities. Their utilization in health plans such as Humana shows effectiveness over time in tailoring interventions to the population. A tool like this would require policymaker and clinician involvement to garner support for incorporating health equity interventions in daily practice.

Another recommendation for equity measurement is the careful consideration of the most appropriate reference group and even whether a comparison is needed to make the main point. Although there is no right or wrong choice of a "reference population," its choice can help with the interpretation of results. From the perspective of the goal of best health for all, choosing the healthiest population as the reference group usually makes sense. For example, if patients who identify as Black are experiencing higher rates of maternal mortality than patients who identify as White, Asian, or Hispanic, it may be compelling to choose non-Black patients as the reference population. However, the case for reducing maternal mortality among Black birthing persons is likely sufficiently compelling as to not require a comparison to an advantaged group.

A widely debated issue is whether the measure of equity should be risk-adjusted [43–45]. That is, whether measures/metrics should analytically control for baseline risk factors associated with outcomes used to measure quality. For both overall and stratified measures/metrics, critics of risk adjustment are concerned that such measures/metrics may understate equity issues, especially when the adjusted factors reflect social disadvantage at the individual, institutional, or community level and represent barriers to access to, effective interaction with, and delivery of healthcare. Adjustments also may implicitly set different standards for patients with different levels and recommend developing a conceptual model on how social and other risk factors relate to the measured outcome to guide variable selection, while considering the constraints of data availability and data quality [46].

Moving from Measurement to Action

Healthcare organizations in the United States are working to create and implement the infrastructures needed to measure, report, and react to the equity of care that they are delivering to different subpopulations of patients. Infrastructure needs for health equity measurement include measurement expertise, data systems to collect, monitor, and convert measures to knowledge and action, and clinician and staff training in data collection, reporting, interpretation, and use in practice. There has been a renewed focus on capturing key sociodemographic data from patients including the patient's race, ethnicity, gender, sexual orientation, and disability status. This work has included training (or retraining) staff on "best practices" for capturing these data, including self-identification by the patient of their own characteristics. Healthcare organizations are then using these sociodemographic data to stratify their quality and safety data, to better understand where disparities or differences might exist in the quality of care delivered to different patient subpopulations and where quality improvement efforts could help close any identified gaps [47].

It is important not only to develop good measures, but we must also attend to how measures are used in research and practice. Health system leaders, healthcare and public health practitioners, policymakers, and researchers must consider how to apply an equity lens to data investigation and reporting. Among the important principles for conducting equity work are practicing routine bias self-checks and peer-checks and seeking to earn and deserve the trust of the study populations by engaging the population that is the subject of the data measurement and the research. In analysis and reporting, we must look for positive as well as negative effects on disadvantaged groups to appreciate the strengths of populations facing historical discrimination. A critical guiding light is being wary of overly simple or simplifying explanations. Health system leaders, healthcare and public health practitioners, policymakers, and researchers must delve into both establishing that differences exist among various subpopulations and explaining why gaps exist, without shying away from structural and cultural complicity in health inequities.

As we select an equity measure to evaluate the achievement of the aims for high-quality care, we must consider whether the measure fits the context and comes from a reliable source. In such investigations, we might ask what is the meaning of race or ethnicity as a variable. Does a binary measure reflect a person's experience? As a social construction that brings along the impact of centuries of racism, in the case of a race or ethnicity measure, researchers must decide whether a variable is responsive to the research question, whether it is appropriately measured, and what the meaning of a difference in the variable between groups is (e.g., is it due to allowable factors, unallowable factors, and is there evidence of social injustice?). Finally, what other measures, such as social determinants of health, must also be considered when seeking to explain specific outcomes?

The lack of concrete resolution of inequitable care in the United States, as noted in the NHQDR [19], raises the important question of whether policymakers should consider financially incentivizing care practices tailored to improve care equity. Through value-based purchasing programs, funders could require organizations to set goals for equity achievement and collect and report performance measures to evaluate progress toward the goals. Measures themselves should be chosen with attention to all available guidance, to be as robust and compelling as possible. An important consideration is whether incentives for meeting equity goals should be structured as upside-only (e.g., bonuses) or whether there should also be losses to organizations failing to meet goals. A problem with other value-based purchasing programs has been their regressive nature – that is, organizations with fewer resources are penalized for not meeting goals, which in turn increases the difficulty of reaching the goals in ensuing rounds. The Center for Medicare and Medicaid Innovation's ACO Realizing Equity, Access, and Community Health (ACO REACH) model hopes to promote progressive value-based payment [44, 48].

Summary and Conclusions

A range of available measurement approaches exists to assess the presence of equity in the delivery of healthcare and the achievement of health outcomes in the United States. Among the most compelling developments in recent years are the notions of "allowable versus unallowable" portions of quality gaps among different groups, using appropriate sources/respondents (e.g., self-report) in assigning demographic characteristics, longitudinal tracking of change over time, and consideration of whether risk adjustment reveals or underestimates healthcare inequity. Fundamentally, the highest quality of care cannot be realized when disparities exist among subgroups of the population, and our achievement of equitable health must be measured to be estimated and to hold policymakers, health system leaders, and health professionals accountable to the populations they serve.

Discussion Questions

9.1 What challenges exist in collecting, standardizing, and sharing demographic data (e.g., race, ethnicity, socioeconomic status) for health equity measurement, and how can health systems address these challenges to ensure equitable care?

9.2 Should health equity measures be risk-adjusted, especially when baseline social disadvantages might reflect systemic inequities? What are the potential risks and benefits of using risk adjustment in equity metrics?

9.3 How can health equity measurement frameworks better account for intersectionality (e.g., race and gender combined) to capture nuanced disparities across multiple social identities?

9.4 How should equity be incorporated into value-based purchasing? Should incentives be structured with upside-only rewards or penalties for failing to meet equity goals? What are the potential implications for under-resourced healthcare organizations?

References

1 Penman-Aguilar, A., Talih, M., Huang, D. et al. (2016). Measurement of health disparities, health inequities, and social determinants of health to support the advancement of health equity. *J. Public Health Manag. Pract.* 22 (Suppl 1): S33–S42. https://doi.org/10.1097/PHH.0000000000000373.

2 Frieden, T.R. (2013). CDC health disparities and inequalities report—United States, 2013. *MMWR Surveill. Summ.* 62 (Suppl 3): 1–2.

3 Braveman, P. (2014). What are health disparities and health equity? We need to be clear. *Public Health Rep.* 129 (Suppl 2): 5–8. https://doi.org/10.1177/00333549141291S203.

4 Duran, D.G. and Pérez-Stable, E.J. (2019). Novel approaches to advance minority health and health disparities research. *Am J Public Health* 109 (S1): S8–S10. https://doi.org/10.2105/ajph.2018.304931.

5 Gourevitch, M.N. (2014). Population health and the academic medical center: the time is right. *Acad. Med.* 89 (4): 544–549.

6 Purnell, T.S., Fakunle, D.O., Bone, L.R. et al. (2019). Overcoming barriers to sustaining health equity interventions: insights from the National Institutes of Health Centers for Population Health and Health Disparities. *J Health Care Poor Underserved.* 30 (3): 1212–1236. https://doi.org/10.1353/hpu.2019.0083.

7 Institute of Medicine (US) Committee on Quality of Health Care in America (2001). *Crossing the Quality Chasm: A New Health System for the 21st Century.* Washington, DC: National Academies Press (US).

8 Agency for Healthcare Research and Quality (2022). Six domains of healthcare quality. Rockville, MD. https://www.ahrq.gov/talkingquality/measures/six-domains.html.

9 Institute of Medicine (US) Committee on Understanding and Eliminating Racial and Ethnic Disparities in Health Care; Smedley, B.D., Stith, A.Y., and Nelson, A.R. (eds.) (2003). *Unequal Treatment: Confronting Racial and Ethnic Disparities in Health Care.* Washington, DC: National Academies Press (US). https://www.ncbi.nlm.nih.gov/books/NBK220358/. https://doi.org/10.17226/12875.

10 Agency for Healthcare Research and Quality (2024). 2023 National Healthcare Quality and Disparities Report. Rockville, MD. https://www.ahrq.gov/research/findings/nhqrdr/nhqdr23/index.html.

11 National Academies of Sciences, Engineering, and Medicine (2024). *Ending Unequal Treatment: Strategies to Achieve Equitable Health Care and Optimal Health for All*. Washington, DC: The National Academies Press. https://doi.org/10.17226/27820.

12 James, C.V., Haley, J.M., Allen, E.H., and Nelson, T. (2023). Using race and ethnicity data to advance health equity: examples, promising practices, remaining challenges, and next steps. The Urban Institute. https://www.urban.org/sites/default/files/2023-10/Using%20Race%20and%20Ethnicity%20Data%20to%20Advance%20Health%20Equity.pdf.

13 Cooper-Patrick, L., Gallo, J.J., Gonzales, J.J. et al. (1999). Race, gender, and partnership in the patient-physician relationship. *JAMA*. 282 (6): 583–589. https://doi.org/10.1001/jama.282.6.583.

14 King, W.D., Wong, M.D., Shapiro, M.F. et al. (2004). Does racial concordance between HIV-positive patients and their physicians affect the time to receipt of protease inhibitors? *J. Gen. Intern. Med.* 19 (11): 1146–1153. https://doi.org/10.1111/j.1525-1497.2004.30443.x.

15 Traylor, A.H., Schmittdiel, J.A., Uratsu, C.S. et al. (2010). Adherence to cardiovascular disease medications: does patient-provider race/ethnicity and language concordance matter? *J. Gen. Intern. Med.* 25 (11): 1172–1177. https://doi.org/10.1007/s11606-010-1424-8.

16 Cooper, L.A., Roter, D.L., Johnson, R.L. et al. (2003). Patient-centered communication, ratings of care, and concordance of patient and physician race. *Ann. Intern. Med.* 139 (11): 907–915. https://doi.org/10.7326/0003-4819-139-11-200312020-00009.

17 Saha, S., Taggart, S.H., Komaromy, M., and Bindman, A.B. (2000). Do patients choose physicians of their own race? *Health Aff (Millwood)*. 19 (4): 76–83.

18 National Institute on Minority Health and Health Disparities (2017). NIMHD research framework. https://nimhd.nih.gov/researchFramework (accessed 3 April 2024).

19 Report of the Secretary's Task Force on Black and Minority Health: The Heckler Report (1985). U.S. Department of Health and Human Services Office of Minority Health.

20 Office of Disease Prevention and Health Promotion (n.d.). Diabetes. Healthy People 2030. U.S. Department of Health and Human Services. https://health.gov/healthypeople/objectives-and-data/browse-objectives/diabetes.

21 National Committee for Quality Assurance (2018). HEDIS measures and technical resources. https://www.ncqa.org/hedis/measures/.

22 Braveman, P., Arkin, E., Orleans, T. et al. (2018). What is health equity? *Behav. Sci. Policy* 4 (1): 1–14.

23 Agency for Healthcare Research and Quality (n.d.). Disparities. https://www.ahrq.gov/topics/disparities.html.

24 McGuire, T.G., Alegria, M., Cook, B.L. et al. (2006). Implementing the Institute of Medicine definition of disparities: an application to mental health care. *Health Serv. Res.* 41 (5): 1979–2005. https://doi.org/10.1111/j.1475-6773.2006.00583.x.

25 Clemans-Cope, L., Garrett, B., McMorrow, S. (2023). How should we measure and interpret racial and ethnic disparities in health care? *Urban Institute and the Robert Wood Johnson Foundation*. https://www.urban.org/sites/default/

files/2023-01/How%20Should%20We%20Measure%20and%20Interpret%20Racial%20and%20Ethnic%20Disparities%20in%20Health%20Care.pdf.

26 Agniel, D., Cabreros, I., Damberg, C.L. et al. (2023). A formal framework for incorporating equity into health care quality measurement. *Health Aff. (Millwood).* 42 (10): 1383–1391. https://doi.org/10.1377/hlthaff.2022.01483.

27 Office of the Assistant Secretary for Planning and Evaluation (2021). Developing Health Equity Measures. U.S. Department of Health and Human Services. https://aspe.hhs.gov/reports/developing-health-equity-measures (accessed 4 April 2024).

28 National Centers for Quality Assurance (2021). Evolution of multicultural health care distinction to health equity accreditation. https://www.ncqa.org/wp-content/uploads/2021/02/20210609_Public_Comment_Overview_MHC_Distinction_Evolving_to_Health_Equity_Accreditation.pdf (accessed 4 April 2024).

29 Cunningham, B.A., Marsteller, J.A., Romano, M.J. et al. (2014). Perceptions of health system orientation: quality, patient centeredness, and cultural competency. *Med. Care Res. Rev.* 71 (6): 559–579. https://doi.org/10.1177/1077558714557891.

30 National Quality Forum (2012). Healthcare disparities and cultural competency consensus standards: disparities-sensitive measurement assessment. https://www.qualityforum.org/Publications/2012/11/Healthcare_Disparities_and_Cultural_Competency_Consensus_Standards__Disparities-Sensitive_Measure_Assessment.aspx.

31 CMS OMH Mapping Medicare Disparities Tool (2024). Center for Medicare and Medicaid services. https://www.cms.gov/priorities/health-equity/minority-health/research-data/mapping-medicare-disparities-tool-mmd.

32 Centers for Medicare & Medicaid Services (2021). Trends in racial, ethnic, sex, and rural-urban inequities in health care in Medicare beneficiaries: 2009–2018. https://www.cms.gov/priorities/health-equity/minority-health/research-data/stratified-reporting.

33 Minnesota Department of Health Center (2022). Eliminating Health disparities initiative: fiscal years 2021 and 2022, report to the Minnesota legislature. https://www.health.state.mn.us/communities/equity/reports.

34 CMS Office of Minority Health in Collaboration with the RAND Corporation (2023). Disparities in health care in Medicare advantage associated with dual eligibility or eligibility for a low-income subsidy and disability. https://www.cms.gov/files/document/2023-disparities-health-care-medicare-advantage-associated-dual-eligibility-or-eligibility-low.pdf.

35 Measures Management System Resource, Centers for Medicare & Medicaid Services (2023). Supporting material for "from data to action: how CMS and stakeholders are addressing inequalities in health care". https://mmshub.cms.gov/sites/default/files/PW-QA-Summary.pdf.

36 Beckett, M.K., Hambarsoomian, K., Martino, S.C. et al. (2023). Measuring equity in the hospital setting: an HCAHPS application of the Health Equity Summary Score. *Med. Care* 61 (1): 3–9. https://doi.org/10.1097/MLR.0000000000001769.

37 Zimmerman, F.J. (2019). A robust health equity metric. *Public Health.* 175: https://doi.org/10.1016/j.puhe.2019.06.008.

38 Zimmerman, F.J. and Anderson, N.W. (2019). Trends in health equity in the United States by race/ethnicity, sex, and income, 1993–2017 [published correction appears in JAMA Netw Open. 2019 Jul 3; 2(7): e199357]. *JAMA Netw. Open* 2 (6): e196386. https://doi.org/10.1001/jamanetworkopen.2019.6386.

39 National Committee for Quality Assurance (2023). Measuring health equity: a review of scoring approaches. https://www.ncqa.org/wp-content/uploads/2023/02/NCQA-MeasuringHealthEquity-Whitepaper-FINAL_WEB.pdf (accessed 4 April 2024).

40 Kindig, D., Lardinois, N., Asada, Y., and Mullahy, J. (2018). Considering mean and inequality health outcomes together: the population health performance index. *Int. J. Equity Health* 17 (1): 25. https://doi.org/10.1186/s12939-018-0731-2.

41 Russell, K.S., Ma, S., Siddiqui, M., and Olayiwola, J.N. (2022). Building the foundation for reducing disparities in Medicare advantage. *NEJM Catalyst* 10. https://doi.org/10.1056/CAT.22.0068.

42 The Leapfrog Group (2024). Leapfrog hospital survey: overview of content for hospitals and stakeholders. https://www.leapfroggroup.org/survey-materials/survey-overview (accessed 4 April 2024).

43 Brook, R.H., Iezzoni, L.I., Jencks, S.F. et al. (1987). Symposium: case-mix measurement and assessing quality of hospital care. *Health Care Financ. Rev.* 24: 39–48.

44 Fiscella, K., Burstin, H.R., and Nerenz, D.R. (2014). Quality measures and sociodemographic risk factors: to adjust or not to adjust. *JAMA.* 312 (24): 2615–2616. https://doi.org/10.1001/jama.2014.15372.

45 Braithwaite, R.S. (2018). Risk adjustment for quality measures is neither binary nor mandatory. *JAMA* 319 (20): 2077–2078.

46 National Quality Forum (2022). Risk adjustment technical guidance final report - Phase 2. https://www.qualityforum.org/Publications/2022/12/Risk_Adjustment_Technical_Guidance_Final_Report_-_Phase_2.aspx.

47 Casey Lion, K., Faro, E.Z., and Coker, T.R. (2022). All quality improvement is health equity work: designing improvement to reduce disparities. *Pediatrics* 149 (Supplement 3): e2020045948E. https://doi.org/10.1542/peds.2020-045948E.

48 Gondi, S., Joynt Maddox, K., and Wadhera, R.K. (2022). "REACHing" for equity - moving from regressive toward progressive value-based payment. *N. Engl. J. Med.* 387 (2): 97–99. https://doi.org/10.1056/NEJMp2204749.

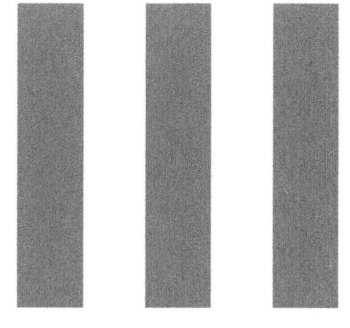

How Do We Use Quality Measurement to Drive Change in Healthcare?

10 Using Performance Data to Drive Improvement and Better Outcomes

Robert Lloyd[1] and Jeffrey Salvon-Harman[2]

[1]*Improvement Science and Methods, Institute for Healthcare Improvement, Boston, MA, USA*

[2]*Safety, Institute for Healthcare Improvement, Boston, MA, USA*

Introduction

Healthcare professionals use a variety of quality improvement (QI) concepts, methods, and tools to understand their systems and provide better care. The general concept is that a health system, healthcare facility, or practice will measure a particular process or outcome, and that the resulting data will be used to drive QI priorities and efforts. QI efforts may include interventions to standardize a process (e.g., implementing an evidence-based guideline) or implement a new structure (e.g., improving the ratio of nurses to patients) to reduce variation and achieve better results and outcomes. Yet, many struggle with an essential aspect of QI – creating effective QI data systems that assess a process or outcome, monitor it over time, and accurately determine whether it has or has not improved. Data systems for QI purposes are different from data systems for financial performance, medical records, or clinical research. This chapter provides an overview of key QI data methods and tools, clarifies the differences between data and information, and presents key issues related to using data to achieve better outcomes.

The Concept of Transparency

When shopping for a new car, online reviews report on the reliability, longevity, and repair records for every car on the market. Similar data exist for hotels, restaurants, vacation home rentals, and airlines. Historically, however, readily available data on the performance of healthcare systems have been lagging. While data have become increasingly available on doctors, hospitals, and health systems' performance, the reliability, timeliness, and representativeness of these data have frequently been called into question. The primary question many consumers and purchasers ask about healthcare data being reported to the public is, *"Why isn't comparative healthcare data more representative of actual patient experiences, outcomes and, more recent?"* The hesitancy of healthcare providers to provide process and outcome data comparable to what is found in other industries comes from decades of secrecy and concealment that has historically received few challenges. This is now changing as patients, payers, and consumer groups are demanding greater transparency.

As we consider greater healthcare transparency, however, a dialogue is needed around three key topics [1]:

- Transparency of what?
- Transparency for whom?
- Transparency at what level?

Assessing organizational transparency is the first step to initiating this dialogue within healthcare organizations. Table 10.1 presents a Transparency Assessment Tool that evaluates perceptions about the frequency of reporting for hospital outcomes, clinical and financial performance, and individual provider performance on key performance indicators [1].

The transparency issue will become even more important as healthcare costs continue to rise and as care delivery continues to be inequitably distributed across populations. Organizations need to become proactive and engaged in transparency, whether extrinsically motivated through required programs by the government or other entities (e.g., payers) or intrinsically motivated through local efforts aimed at improving specific processes that demonstrate their vision and mission statements. The best approach is to understand performance data and its limitations, as well as the requirements for programs where the data from an organization can be used for public reporting, pay for performance, or quality assessment.

Drivers of Improvement in Healthcare Organizations and Systems

Improving healthcare performance is driven by both intrinsic and extrinsic factors. Professionally and altruistically, clinicians and the healthcare workforce are intrinsically motivated to provide the highest quality and

Table 10.1: Transparency Assessment Tool.

Level and frequency of transparency	Strongly agree	Agree	Not sure	Disagree	Strongly disagree
1. Greater transparency is needed across all healthcare settings and providers.					
2. Patients should be able to compare hospitals as easily as they do cars and other products.					
3. Results on hospital outcomes (mortality, infections, falls, med errors, etc.) should be made public *once a year*.					
4. Results on hospital outcomes (mortality, infections, falls, med errors, etc.) should be made public *twice a year*.					
5. Results on hospital outcomes (mortality, infections, falls, med errors, etc.) should be made public *four times a year*.					
6. Results on groups of doctors (surgeons, GPs, intensivists, dentists, etc.) should be made public *once a year*.					
7. Results on individual doctors should be made public *once a year*.					
8. All clinical outcomes on hospital performance should be made available to the public.					
9. Operational outcomes on hospital performance (wait times, referral times, and access) should be made available to the public.					
10. Patient satisfaction results for each hospital should be made available to the public.					
11. Financial results (including salaries) for each hospital should be made available to the public.					
12. Mortality rates for individual surgeons should be made available to the public.					
13. Infection rates for individual physicians should be made available to the public.					

(Continued)

Table 10.1: (Continued)

Level and frequency of transparency	Strongly agree	Agree	Not sure	Disagree	Strongly disagree
14. Errors and harm rates for individual physicians should be made available to the public.					
15. Salaries of individual physicians should be made available to the public.					

Source: Reproduced from Lloyd [1] / Jones & Bartlett Learning.

safest care. The desire to help others drew most of the workforce into the healing professions. The fiduciary relationship between clinicians and patients [2] – driven by the Hippocratic Oath and stemming from the trust relationship in which the physician acts or advises in the patient's best interest – is another intrinsic motivator for self-assessing performance through data and engaging in steps to improve care. In the context of (1) productivity pressures, (2) increasing demand for services, and (3) the increasing complexity of medical care and its delivery, influences intrinsic to an organization that demonstrate improved performance, both clinically and operationally, need to emerge and evolve.

Leaders of healthcare systems need to create strategic quality, safety, and experience goals for the entire organization and ensure those goals are communicated to all members of the workforce for alignment of improvement efforts. Whether created by the organization's governing board(s) or leadership team, these motivational factors cascade to frontline leaders overseeing care delivery by clinical professionals. Frontline leaders may also create data-driven targets (e.g., percentage of patients receiving broad-spectrum antimicrobials over extended periods) in pursuit of the overarching organizational goals (e.g., strategic goal to eliminate preventable harm from *Clostridioides difficile* colitis). All these influences span from individual to organizational intrinsic factors.

Regulatory, accreditation entities, and payors, as well as business and consumer groups, play an extrinsic role in driving healthcare improvement through their standards, goals, and targets, which are based on quality, safety, and cost. Regulators like the Centers for Medicare & Medicaid Services (CMS) seek to assure the public that care is being delivered in a manner consistent with standards of care and professional guidelines. Organizations like the Joint Commission, which accredits hospitals, evaluate and score organizations as meeting or exceeding observable quality and safety standards. Payors seek to ensure that comparative reference targets of quality in care delivery are met to justify payments for services.

As both intrinsic and extrinsic motivational factors are considered, it is important to acknowledge the research on these topics and which motivational approach has the greatest ability to influence performance. Across many industries, intrinsic motivation exceeds extrinsic motivation for its effect on performance. Within healthcare, intrinsic motivation is confirmed to increase performance, engagement, and meaning [3]. So, in this context, QI efforts should be inspired, and similarly sustained, by tapping into the intrinsic motivators of healthcare professionals (e.g., quality of care outcomes, safety of care delivery, and patient experience of care).

Finally, consider the predicament of healthcare providers. By their very nature and training, most clinical professionals are focused on improvement. The external perception that they are too busy with clinical duties to engage in QI belies their professional interests in providing the highest quality and safest care for their patients. Arriving from competitive academic and training environments, the use of data for comparability and assessment is not a foreign concept to these individuals. In fact, comparative data provides the foundation for stimulating dialogues and opportunities for learning. The major challenge, however, in using comparative data is when it is used for rating and ranking of healthcare providers and their organizations. Such a focus on data for judgment subverts intrinsic motivation and leads to data for judgment, not data for learning. Thus, healthcare providers today are constantly struggling to balance the inherent intrinsic motivating forces against the more insidious nature of extrinsic motivation.

Approaches to Performance Measurement

The question to ask before ever starting collection and analysis of any data is, why measure? Solberg and colleagues suggest that there are three fundamental approaches to measuring healthcare performance: (1) accountability (i.e., measurement for judgment or rating and rankings), (2) clinical research (e.g., randomized control trials exploring the efficacy of an intervention), or (3) improvement (i.e., measuring process performance over time rather than at fixed points in time) [4]. Many are familiar with accountability data (e.g., CMS Hospital Compare or state data commissions) and clinical research data derived from statistically powered sample populations and the strength of a statistical test of significance between two groups as determined by the p-value. However, fewer are familiar with time series analysis that displays data on run charts or statistical process control (SPC) charts to measure and demonstrate improvement over time, not at two fixed points in time. While all three approaches have a role in evaluating healthcare performance and outcomes, each takes a very different path when it comes to setting an aim or purpose, gathering data, and using statistical testing methods designed to determine if a change has achieved the stated aim. When the aims and methods of the three approaches are intermixed, there is a risk of sending confusing messages to those working in the organization. Additionally, since the conclusions drawn from different statistical methods and techniques used in each of the three approaches fundamentally and operationally differ (e.g., enumerative versus analytic methods and techniques [5]), the same data may in fact produce widely different conclusions. More specifically, because the three measurement approaches employ different methods and statistical techniques, it is very likely that conclusions drawn from the data that are aimed at judgment and accountability can erode psychological safety and willingness to engage in improvement efforts.

Designing a Data Collection Plan

Is it data or information that is needed?

> *Data refers to the raw facts and figures which are collected as part of the normal functioning of the hospital. Information, on the other hand, is defined as data, which have been processed and analyzed in a formal, intelligent way, so that the results are directly useful to those involved in the operation and management of the hospital [6].*

The distinction reinforces the fact that data are not information. Data are represented by qualitative and quantitative bits and bytes believed to capture some aspect of reality. Data can be tabulated and analyzed statistically and extracted from a computer. This is the limitation of data. Information, on the other hand, comes not from the computer but is derived when humans place the data and the statistical analyses into a context, test theories, and create meaning. Individuals who can translate data into useful information for decision-making serve a key role in the measurement of organizational priorities and performance. The goal is to use information to test theories and ultimately make improvements.

The collection and analysis of data should be a deliberate journey characterized by both technical and logical milestones. Figure 10.1 provides a roadmap for this journey along with key milestones to guide the way [1]. Several of the milestones deal specifically with data collection: stratification, sampling, and frequency and duration of data collection. Each of these is briefly addressed below (Figure 10.1).

- **Stratification**: This step requires the knowledge of subject matter experts (SMEs) who can describe how a process logically functions and factors that may disrupt a process or create differences in performance. Stratification consists of separating and classifying data into homogeneous categories that reflect common characteristics. The objective of

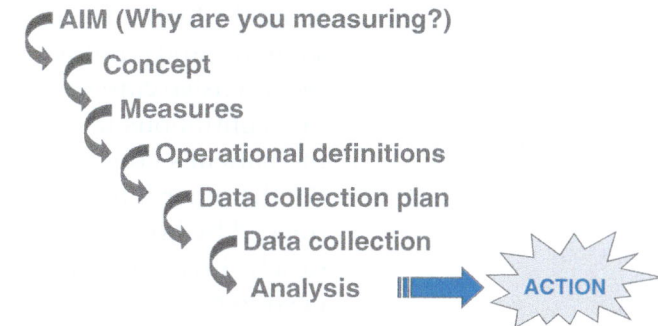

Figure 10.1: Milestones in the quality measurement journey.

Source: Reproduced from Lloyd [1] / with permission of Jones & Bartlett Learning.

stratification is to reduce confounding of the data. Stratification helps create categories of data believed to be mutually exclusive and therefore allows discovery of patterns that would not be otherwise observable. A fundamental principle of statistical analysis is to minimize variation within a group to maximize the comparison of variation between groups. Stratification operationalizes this principle. Typical stratification categories include personal and social determinants, comorbidities, severity, prior admissions, time of day, day of week, shift, or type of procedure. The final consideration about stratification is that it should be designed with the SMEs before collecting data. Once the data have been collected, it is oftentimes a major challenge and time-consuming activity to tease apart the various stratification levels.

- **Sampling**: Sampling may be the single most important action that can reduce the time and resources spent collecting data from large source pools. Ishikawa, in his classic work, *Guide to Quality Control* [7], identified four conditions for developing a sampling plan: accuracy, reliability, speed, and economy. It is nearly impossible to obtain a sample that meets all four criteria simultaneously. Sampling, therefore, consists of compromises and tradeoffs. The key to successful sampling relates to (1) understanding the overall purpose of selecting a sample and (2) the advantages and disadvantages of each specific sampling methodology.

  The primary objective of sampling is to draw a limited number of observations that are representative of the larger population from which the sample is drawn. If the sample is not representative of the population, the risk of deriving erroneous or biased conclusions about the population under study increases.

- **Frequency and Duration of Data Collection**: The frequency of data collection refers to the period in which data are collected (e.g., daily, hourly, and monthly). Duration refers to how long data are to be collected. Is data collected at a single point in time or on a continuous basis? The need to know, the criticality of the measures, and the amount of data required to make conclusions should drive decisions about the frequency and duration of data collection and whether to use sampling and stratification methods. For example, when a patient is in the intensive care unit (ICU), their vital signs are typically monitored in a continuous manner via telemetry. In this case, the criticality of the patient's condition requires moment-to-moment data collection. On the other hand, monitoring cholesterol levels does not need to be tracked by hour, day, or week since it is a marker that changes more slowly. Frequency and duration of data collection, therefore, always need to be placed within the context of the need to know.

Understanding Variation Conceptually

Organizations committed to making quality their organization's operating strategy need to ensure that leaders, managers, and staff all understand variation conceptually and statistically – a central theme articulated in Dr. Deming's classic works, *Out of the Crisis* and *The New Economics* [8, 9]. In a healthcare context, Dr. Don Berwick described the critical role of understanding variation conceptually and statistically in "Controlling Variation in Healthcare: A Consultation from Walter Shewhart [10]." Yet, despite these foundational references, a pervasive challenge in healthcare has been the steadfast use of aggregated data and summary statistics for sensemaking of the data. This leads to a tendency to compare, for example, this quarter's length of stay (LOS) in the ICU with last quarter's LOS. Such comparisons usually lead to using data for accountability or judgment rather than improvement. When this happens, leaders will judge whether performance at a specific point in time is acceptable or unacceptable. This binomial approach to decision-making limits insights into whether performance is improving or worsening over time. Dr. Myron Tribus wrote that, "*Managing a company by means of the monthly (or quarterly or yearly) report is like trying to drive a car by watching the yellow line in the rear-view mirror* [11]." The meaningful alternative to looking at data from a static and/or retrospective viewpoint is to take a dynamic approach and look at the data over time. Time series analysis is at the center of understanding variation for QI. Returning to the ICU example, clinicians are observing the variation in the patient's vital signs over time, not averaging diastolic and systolic blood pressure readings over time. Improving clinical outcomes requires tracking data over time, not in the aggregate. Similar thinking should guide all QI efforts.

Analyzing variation conceptually requires knowledge of two key concepts: **common cause variation** and **special cause variation** [12]. Table 10.2 provides a summary of the key characteristics of each form of variation. Common cause variation characterizes a stable and therefore predictable process. This does not mean, however, that the process performance is acceptable or desired. Shewhart summarized common cause variation as follows: "*A phenomenon will be said to be controlled when, through the use of past experience, we can predict, at least within limits, how the phenomenon may be expected to*

Table 10.2: Characteristics of common and special cause variation.

Common cause variation	Special cause variation
▪ Is inherent in the design of the process	▪ Is due to irregular or unnatural causes that are not inherent in the design of the process
▪ Is due to regular, natural, or ordinary causes	▪ Affect some, but not necessarily all, aspects of the process
▪ Affects all the outcomes of a process	▪ Results in an "unstable" process that is not predictable
▪ Results in a "stable" process that is predictable	▪ Also known as non-random or assignable variation
▪ Also known as random or unassignable variation	

Source: Reproduced from Lloyd [1] / with permission of Jones & Bartlett Learning.

vary in the future [12]." From a clinical perspective, a patient might have a systolic blood pressure that averages 175 mm Hg with a spread of 165–185 mm Hg. In this case, the patient's systolic blood pressure is stable and predictable but is unacceptably elevated.

Special cause variation, on the other hand, results from irregular or unnatural causes that are not inherent in the normal functioning of a process. The presence of a special cause is a signal that the performance of the process is unstable and not predictable. For example, the patient on telemetry in the ICU displays stable monitor readings within acceptable parameters over a period (i.e., common cause variation). But if the patient's blood pressure is now observed to be lower than the acceptable specification limit, this would constitute a special cause. When faced with a special cause, such as low blood pressure, the correct action is to investigate why the patient's blood pressure has transitioned from a common cause to a special cause state.

The final consideration for addressing special causes is to extricate the reasons why a special cause occurred. If the factors that led to a special cause (e.g., a medication error) are not extricated from the process, then there is a very high probability that the special cause will recur at some point in the future. Reason uses the term "latent errors" to describe special causes that go unaddressed and have a high probability of recurring [13].

Understanding Variation Statistically

Once variation is understood conceptually, it is time to build skills in understanding variation statistically. This is where SPC concepts, methods, and tools come into the picture. SPC is a branch of analytic statistics that uses

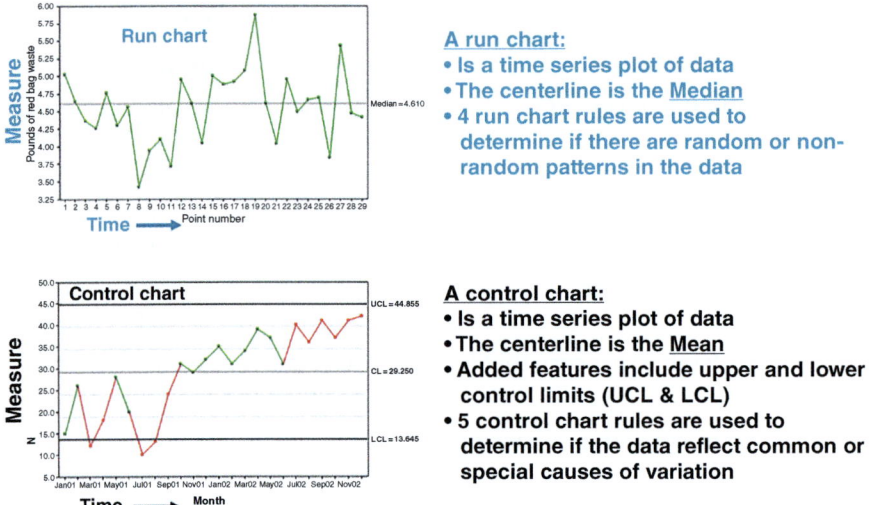

Figure 10.2: The two key tools for analyzing variation.

Source: Reproduced from Lloyd [1] / with permission of Jones & Bartlett Learning.

time series analysis to understand the variation in a process over time [5, 14]. Two key statistical tools are used in this regard: the run chart and Shewhart (control) charts. Figure 10.2 summarizes the characteristics of these two essential QI tools.

Most QI projects begin with a run chart. When constructing a run chart, any type of data can be placed on the chart (e.g., counts, volumes, percentages, scores, and rates). Once the median is placed on the chart as the center line, the next step is to apply four run chart rules to determine if the chart displays random or non-random variation. When using Shewhart charts, however, more knowledge is required. Compared to the one basic way to construct a run chart, there are many options available for constructing Shewhart charts. In healthcare QI work, five different types of Shewhart charts will meet a majority of a QI team's analytic needs (see Figure 10.3). Selecting the appropriate chart for the measures begins by determining the type of data collected: variables (i.e., interval or ratio data that is continuous) or attributes (i.e., categorical or classification data). Once these decisions are made, the most appropriate Shewhart chart can be selected and constructed. The analysis step comes next. Five statistical rules can be applied to determine if special causes are present in the data. The details on run charts and Shewhart charts, along with their construction and interpretation, can be found in books by Lloyd and Provost and Murray [1, 15].

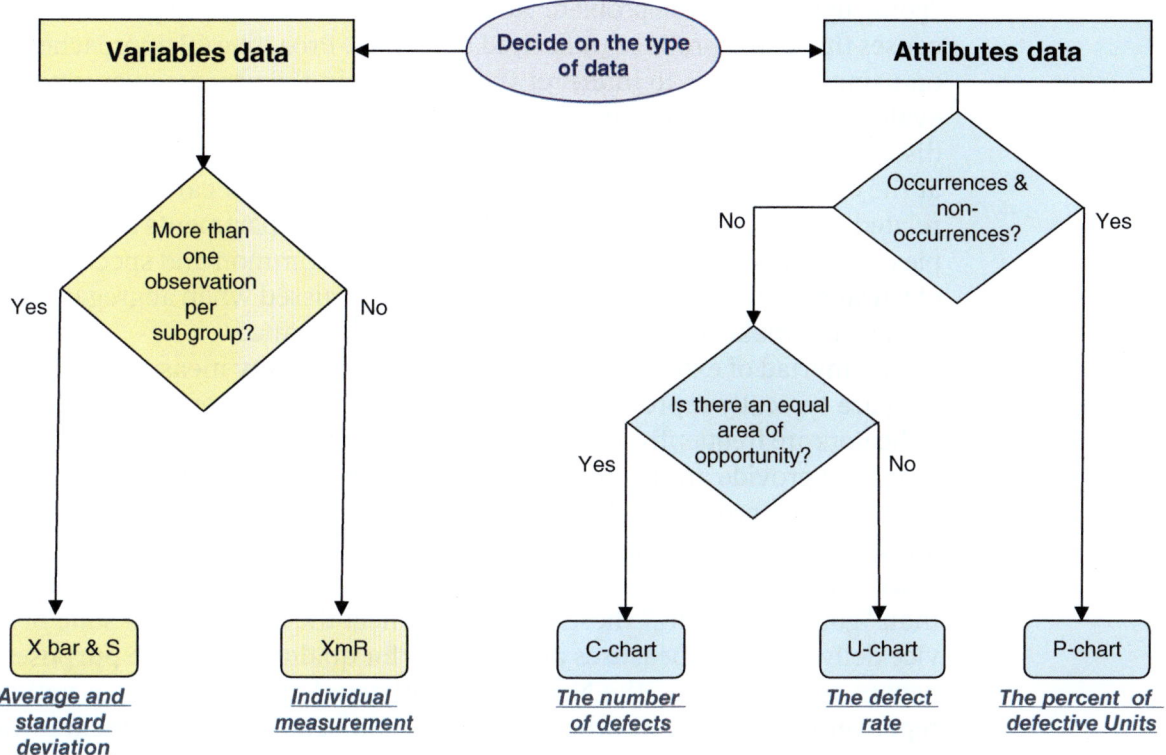

Figure 10.3: The control chart decision tree.

Source: Reproduced from Lloyd [1] / with permission of Jones & Bartlett Learning.

When Should Performance Data Be Used to Drive Improvement and Safety?

Performance data can be placed into a proactive or reactive context. The proactive context relies on using leading indicators of performance, meaning those measurable elements of performance tracked over time that predict expected or desired outcomes and avoidance of undesired outcomes. Leading indicators, however, are not typically the measures reported externally to payors or regulators. Leading indicators are precursor conditions or process variables that are believed to causally drive the outcomes. For example, the number of patients with indwelling urinary catheters remaining in place beyond 48 hours (absent a condition-specific justification) is a leading indicator for catheter-associated urinary tract infection (CAUTI). Not all these patients will develop a CAUTI; however, by removing unnecessary urinary catheters at or before 48 hours, the risk of CAUTI is essentially eliminated entirely [16]. The proactive or causal approach is sometimes referred to as "going upstream of the problem" to address latent factors and prevent special causes that could produce undesired outcomes. Proactive QI approaches rely on using SPC charts to interpret the variation in the process over time (i.e., evaluating the data for common cause or special cause variation). Infectious disease seasonal variation, historical patterns of patients presenting for care at the emergency department, or identifying patterns of care complications related to change of shift across multiple hospital departments are all examples of opportunities to evaluate the presence of common and special causes of variation. These distinct signal types can be missed when aggregated data are used to make decisions about process performance.

The myriad of externally reported quality and safety measures in healthcare are typically represented by lagging indicators of performance. These indicators are frequently aggregated over time (i.e., by month, quarter, or even year) and provide an historical perspective but little insight on the inherent variation in a process and its outcomes. The quality or safety of the system and individual performance are reflected only after services have been provided and there is opportunity to learn after events have occurred. Rather than "going upstream," these measures reflect the downstream state of service delivery. Such measures are reported for quality assurance purposes to payors, registries (e.g., the National Healthcare Safety Network, a national reporting database for healthcare-associated infections, and healthcare workforce communicable infections), and external rating and ranking or recognition programs, among others. Compounding the relative ineffectiveness of lagging indicators for quality and safety control and improvement is the use of averaging the internally selected lagging indicators within healthcare organizations and systems. For example, averages dilute the variation in the process. Furthermore, it is very likely that no single observation is at the average. Half the data could be above the mean and the other half below the mean. Thus, regression to the mean occurs, which eliminates the ability to understand the variation in the process and determine if special causes are present.

An additional leadership and accountability practice that erodes the potential value of measures for QI is the dashboard process that uses "stoplight" indicators for accountability (i.e., the popular red/yellow/green or RYG displays of data). These stoplight visualizations distill useful data over time into single point-in-time indicators of a highly superficial nature. Variation in the data is suppressed when looking at stoplight graphics. No indication of special cause or common cause variation is evident, or even desired, in RYG displays. Therefore, such meaningless rank order analysis should not be used for improvement. Stoplight graphics only lead to using the data for judgment. Unfortunately, healthcare is replete with averaged lagging indicators and stoplight graphics due mainly to the influence of payors, regulators, external recognition programs, and the media. In actuality, leading indicators eclipse the value of lagging indicators for process improvement by identifying opportunities for addressing hazards and risks prior to an undesired outcome occurring. As Donabedian [17, 18] stressed and Berwick reinforced [10], outcomes (lagging variables) will never change unless work focuses on improving the structures and processes (leading indicators) that drive the outcomes. Harping on improving outcomes without working on the structures, processes (and we would add cultures) that causally drive the outcomes will never result in change for the better.

Leading Change of Measurement Strategies

Transforming measurement methods and analytics at the enterprise level can be a herculean endeavor in the absence of effective change management and QI strategies. Change of this magnitude does not lend itself to a "just do it" approach, where the organization can just issue an order to measure and report differently across many workforce segments and amid a history of "doing it the way we've always done it." Change management is the process of building awareness for the needed change ideas, messaged through many channels and tailored to the context of those being asked to change their perspectives and measurement practices. Willingness to participate in or even lead this change is a necessity for those generating, analyzing, and reporting the data. In addition, those responding to the data signals and modifying healthcare service delivery for every patient need to have similar skills. Ideas and the will to execute change often require activation of agency by those with authority within the organization and by those with influence (as informal leaders) [19]. This agency enables co-design of the work processes in response to the signals detected in the data. With a majority of those affected by the change activated, the next steps of introduction and training aimed at building capability for QI throughout the organization can set the stage for testing and implementing a new QI measurement system. Importantly, planning for sustaining changes during the design of the changes is vital for long-term success. Reinforcing the new way of measuring and reporting through substantive use of the measures and sharing improvement successes strengthens the case for making the change in the first place and maintaining the practice to fully realize its promise.

In addition to establishing a QI measurement system, it is important to balance the collection and analysis of quantitative data with qualitative data obtained through storytelling and listening to the voice of the customer. Storytelling brings to life the value and impact of the change in human terms. Translating the level of effort and dollar cost of preventing an adverse event into the human experience of alleviating suffering, increasing quality years of life, improving activities of daily living, and increasing opportunities for participating in personal, family, or community milestones can bring to life the importance of driving QI and better outcomes through the application of meaningful measures and data.

Using the Dosing Approach to Build Organizational Capability for Improvement

Building capability for improvement is not accomplished by requiring staff to attend a "training" session. Organizational capability is a journey that is achieved through an ongoing strategic and tactical commitment to learning and development. A key point in charting a successful learning journey is realizing that not everyone in the organization needs to have the same depth of knowledge in the science of improvement (SOI). "Dosages" of the SOI should vary depending on an individual's role in an organization's quality journey and how much improvement knowledge they need to be effective. Therefore, it is incumbent on the organization's leaders to have a serious dialogue about the dose of the SOI necessary for various roles and individuals within the organization. The dose, for example, that board members and senior leaders need will be different from what middle managers and supervisors need. The dose of the SOI for those delivering care will be different from what supervisors receive, and both doses will be different from the deeper dose that those expected to coach and advise improvement teams should receive. Figure 10.4 provides an example of an organization's completed dosing strategy [1].

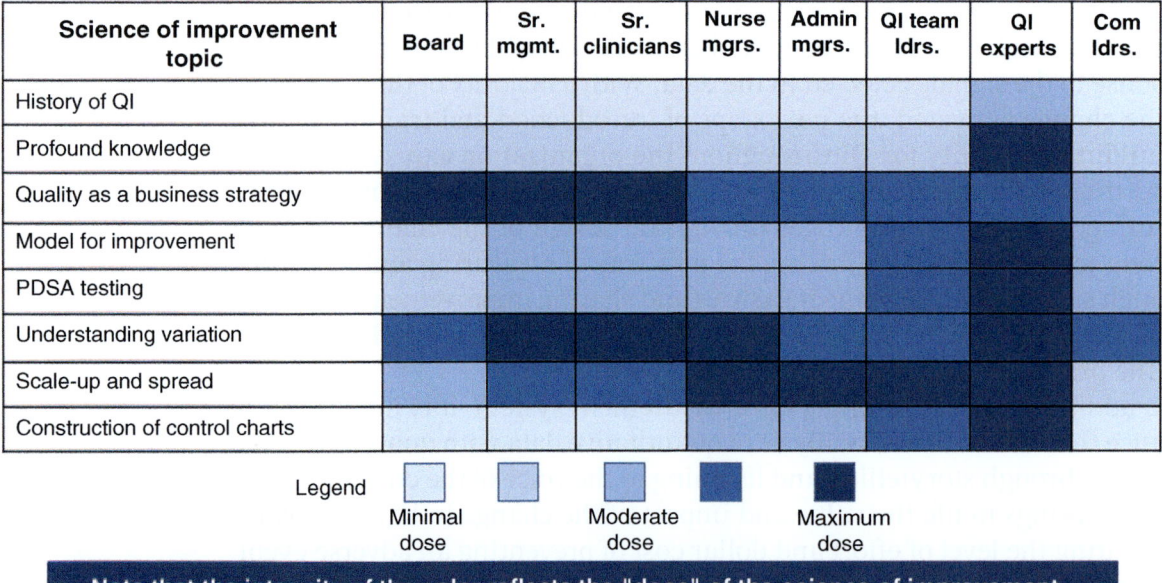

Figure 10.4: Applying the dosing approach to an organization's QI learning plan.

Source: Reproduced from Lloyd [1] / with permission of Jones & Bartlett Learning.

Connecting the Dots

Building a performance measurement system that works is not a difficult strategic task. However, it does require time, systems thinking, and constancy of purpose. As referenced previously, outcomes will never change unless you first work on the structures, processes, and cultures that drive outcomes. This guidance applies not only to individual quality and safety outcomes but also to the bigger challenge of building capacity and capability for improvement throughout the organization. Such system-wide change requires leadership. When Dr. Deming was asked who is responsible for the quality of the organization, he always responded, *"Quality begins with intent, which is fixed by management* [8]." Your quality journey requires systems thinking and constancy of purpose. It can begin today.

Discussion Questions

10.1 What are the benefits and challenges of increasing transparency at different levels (e.g., organizational, individual provider, and public)? How can healthcare organizations balance transparency with concerns about misinterpretation or misuse of data?

10.2 How can healthcare leaders leverage intrinsic motivators to foster sustained QI in their organizations?

10.3 This chapter discusses the importance of shifting from lagging (reactive) indicators to leading (proactive) indicators in performance measurement. Can you think of specific examples in healthcare where leading indicators could be applied effectively? What challenges might arise by analyzing leading indicators over time?

10.4 Distinguishing common cause and special cause variation is central to effective QI. How can healthcare organizations build staff knowledge and capacity to identify and respond to these types of variation? What risks arise when these concepts are misunderstood?

10.5 Implementing a robust QI measurement system often requires cultural and structural change within an organization. What strategies can leaders employ to overcome resistance and build broad support for such changes? How do storytelling and qualitative data contribute to this process?

References

1 Lloyd, R. (2019). *Quality Health Care: A Guide to Developing and Using Indicators*, 2e. Burlington, MA: Jones & Bartlett Learning.

2 Ludewigs, S., Narchi, J., Kiefer, L. et al. (2022). Ethics of the fiduciary relationship between patient and physician: the case of informed consent. *J. Med. Ethics*. https://doi.org/10.1136/jme-2022-108539.

3 Austin, J.M. and Pronovost, P.J. (2016). Improving performance on core processes of care. *Curr. Opin. Allergy Clin. Immunol.* 16 (3): 224–230.

4 Solberg, L., Mosser, G., and McDonald, S. (1997). The three faces of performance measurement: improvement, accountability and research. *Jt. Comm. J. Qual. Improv.* 23 (3): 135–147.

5 Deming, W.E. (1975). On probability as a basis for action. *Am. Stat.* 29 (4): 146–152.

6 Austin, C. (1983). *Information Systems for Hospital Administration*, 24. Chicago, IL: Health Administration Press.

7 Ishikawa, K. (1982). *Guide to Quality Control*. Tokyo: Asian Productivity Organization.

8 Deming, W.E. (1992). *Out of the Crisis*. Cambridge, MA: MIT Press.

9 Deming, W.E. (2000). *The New Economics for Industry, Government, Education*, 2e. Cambridge, MA: MIT Press.

10 Berwick, D.M. (1991). Controlling variation in health care: a consultation from Walter Shewhart. *Med. Care* 29 (12): 1212–1225.

11 Wheeler, D. (1993). *Understanding Variation: The Key to Managing Chaos*, 4. Knoxville, TN: SPC Press, Inc.

12 Shewhart, W.A. (1931). *Economic Control of Quality of Manufactured Product*. New York, NY: D. Van Nostrand Company, Inc.

13 Reason, J. (2000). Human error: models and management. *BMJ* 18 (320): 768–770.

14 Deming, W.E. (1942). On classification of the problems of statistical inference. *J. Am. Stat. Assoc.* 37 (218): 173–185.

15 Provost, L. and Murray, S. (2022). *The Health Care Data Guide*, 2e. San Francisco, CA: Jossey-Bass.

16 Lo, E., Nicolle, L.E., Coffin, S.E. et al. (2014). Strategies to prevent catheter-associated urinary tract infections in acute care hospitals: 2014 update. *Infect. Control Hosp. Epidemiol.* 35 (5): 464–479.

17 Donabedian, A. (1980). *Explorations in Quality Assessment and Monitoring. Vol. 1: The Definition of Quality and Approaches to Its Assessment*. Ann Arbor, MI: Health Administration Press.

18 Donabedian, A. (1982). *Explorations in Quality Assessment and Monitoring. Vol. 2: The Criteria and Standards of Quality*. Ann Arbor, MI: Health Administration Press.

19 Hilton, K. and Anderson, A. (2018). IHI psychology of change framework to advance and sustain improvement. In: *IHI White Paper*. Boston, MA: Institute for Healthcare Improvement. https://www.ihi.org/resources/white-papers/ihi-psychology-change-framework.

11

Integrating Performance Measurement into Payment Policy – The Role of the Federal Government in the United States

Michelle Schreiber and Lee A. Fleisher[1]

[1]University of Pennsylvania Perelman School of Medicine, Duke Margolis Institute for Health Policy, Durham, NC, USA

The United States (US) Federal Government plays a significant role in the use of healthcare quality performance measurement. The Federal Government's goal is to promote accountability through payment and public reporting, to link to national quality improvement efforts, and to provide consumers with usable, transparent data to inform healthcare choices. The Centers for Medicare & Medicaid Services (CMS) has the largest role in the use of quality measurement in payment policy, through its numerous statutory value-based programs (VBPs) and in setting strategic direction. Other agencies also play important roles in the development and use of quality measurement, including the Centers for Disease Control (CDC), the Agency for Healthcare Research and Quality (AHRQ), the Health Resources and Services Administration (HRSA), the Veterans Health Administration (VHA), the military healthcare systems, and others.

CMS is the single largest US payer for healthcare services, covering nearly 150 million persons through its payment programs of Medicare Fee-for-Service (FFS), Medicare Advantage (MA), Marketplace, Innovation Models (CMMI), and Medicaid and Children's Health Insurance Program (CHIP)

Quality Measurement in Healthcare, First Edition. Edited by Jesse M. Pines, Helen Burstin, and Jane Hyatt Thorpe.
© 2025 Jesse M. Pines, Helen Burstin, and Jane Hyatt Thorpe.
Published 2025 by John Wiley & Sons Ltd.

services. Together, these programs account for over $1 trillion in annual healthcare expenditures (nearly 18% of US gross domestic product [GDP]) [1]. Each program has various associated VBPs, which link payment to quality reporting and/or performance in order to promote accountability, transparency, and consumer information [1].

The concept of quality measurement could be linked back to the time of Hippocrates, whose oath incorporated the concept of "first, do no harm." This codified the goal and role of a physician and set an expectation for some measurement. Yet it was not until Dr. Ignaz Semmelweis, a 19th century obstetrician, demonstrated that handwashing reduced maternal mortality during the birth process that data-driven performance measurement began. However, Semmelweis was notably unsuccessful in persuading his colleagues to change their practice – an issue that remains a challenge today [2]. In the 1800s, Florence Nightingale linked poor living conditions and death rates among army soldiers, introducing the use of data and statistics to drive improvement [3]. Ernest Codman pioneered the creation of hospital standards with an emphasis on using data and strategies to address healthcare outcomes in the early 1900s [4].

Quality measurement today has now evolved to include a vast array of stakeholders. These include measure developers, specialty societies, academic organizations, third-party data intermediaries, commercial payers, various quality alliances, healthcare facilities and advocacy groups, multiple federal agencies, companies with a stake in products that may benefit from the use of quality measurement, and others. Quality measurement has proliferated. This, in turn, has led to a re-engineering of some processes in healthcare, identification of key metrics and processes to follow, rewards and penalties for performance, public transparency of performance, and standardized development of quality improvement tools. It has also developed an industry around strategies to maximize a facilities' or group's result on the measure. Nevertheless, a commitment to quality performance, quality improvement, and quality education is now an expectation across healthcare settings. This reaches from the boardroom to front-line staff and influences healthcare education [5]. Although there are both pros and cons to this focus on metrics, especially within payment programs, there is no doubt that the highest quality, safest, and most equitable care should be healthcare's mission and that metrics are essential in understanding progress.

History of the Use of Quality Measurement Across CMS Value-Based Programs

Quality measures are used in multiple CMS VBPs to drive accountability and transparency. In 1965 Congress established the Medicare and Medicaid programs as Title XVIII and Title XIX of the Social Security Act. Within these statutes, Congress also established a set of "Conditions of Participation," which sets forth requirements for several quality elements of hospitals to be eligible for Medicare and Medicaid payment. These included staff credentialing, 24-hour nursing services, and utilization review. The Conditions of Participation established the first quality monitoring programs that relied on metrics. To further advance quality review, in 1972, Congress established the beginnings of the care review organizations – physician-led organizations funded by the National Center for Health Services Research (which became AHRQ). The first care review organizations had the authority and responsibility to review the quality and appropriateness of healthcare delivery in inpatient and outpatient settings. The findings of their quality reviews were linked to improvement strategies.

Medicare's Professional Standards Review Organizations (PSROs) evolved into Peer Review Organizations (PROs) that also included a focus on validating diagnosis-related groups (DRG) – which are used to assign diagnoses to hospital admissions. They also focused on decreasing admissions and readmissions, reducing complications and mortality, and ensuring best practices. PROs were also given the authority to review care and develop medical education requirements, disciplinary actions, and review Medicare billing practices. Many PROs were state-based and physician-led. They have evolved over time to focus on quality improvement. In 1982 the PROs changed their name to Quality Improvement Organizations (QIO) as they are recognized today. Congress authorized the QIO program in 1982 through Title XI and XVIII of the Social Security Act. An expectation for following standards also remains through the guidance, survey, and Conditions of Participation as well as associated and expanded audit and review processes. These government programs were also supplemented by the efforts of each hospital staff, local and state agencies, and organizational and academic medicine, which supported research to develop evidence-based practices.

CMS VBP began as early as 2003 with the Medicare Modernization Act (MMA), which established the Inpatient Quality Reporting Program. The Deficit Reduction Act of 2005 (DRA) introduced potential payment reductions for certain safety events, primarily those that were hospital-based. In 2008, the Medicare Improvements for Patients and Providers (MIPPA) established the first program to directly link payment to quality performance for end-stage renal disease (ESRD) (dialysis) facilities. In 2009, the Consensus-Based Entity (for measures review) was funded based on modifications to the law, Social Security Act (SSA) § 1890A, enacted in MIPPA. The Consensus-Based Entity – which for many years was the National Quality Forum and was transitioned to Batelle Memorial Institute in 2023 – assembles groups of stakeholders to review, give feedback on, and provide recommendations for measures for public and private programs. The 2010 Patient Protection and Accountable Care Act (PPACA, often referred to as ACA) significantly expanded the development of multiple VBPs, including the Hospital VBP (HVBP), the Hospital Readmissions Reduction Program (HRPP), Hospital Acquired Conditions (HAC), and the Skilled Nursing Facilities (SNF)

Quality Reporting Program (QRP). It also established the innovation model program of CMMI, the Qualified Health Plan (QHP) Marketplace quality ratings, the Inpatient Psychiatric program quality reporting program, and the Prospective Cancer Hospital Quality Reporting Program. These programs developed over subsequent years, and many were implemented between 2012 and 2015. The Improving Medicare Post-Acute Care Transformation (IMPACT) Act of 2014 extended more VBPs across post-acute care facilities (SNF, Long-term Care hospitals [LTCH], Home Health [HH], Inpatient Rehabilitation Facility [IRF]), and mandated an aligned approach to PAC quality reporting via patient assessment instruments. Subsequently, newer VBPs include the SNF VBP (in addition to the quality reporting program), the national expansion of the CMMI model HH VBP (in addition to the quality reporting program), and the rural emergency hospitals (REH) quality reporting program.

An important feature of Medicare VBP has been the mix of incentives and penalties related to performance in Medicare payment of up to 9% in the Merit-Based Incentive Payment System (MIPS) program. Because most programs have modest incentives and penalties, concerns have been raised about whether they are adequate for organizations to dedicate resources to changing performance [6]. The potential "costs" of the extra work may be weighed against any potential financial benefit by the providers in determining how much attention is focused on quality programs.

In addition to VBPs noted above, CMS expanded its public reporting programs and initiated the "Stars" programs. The Stars program consolidates performance information into a 1 (poor performance) to 5 rating (excellent performance), which is intended to make the ratings understandable for consumers. In our experience, public reporting of quality measures and the Stars programs may be more effective than the limited incentives/penalties in VBP to drive the organizational change required to improve quality metrics. Many health systems publicly display their rankings on quality programs. Additionally, commercial insurers can link programs to federal ratings. Public reporting is found through the Care Compare website, which reports on performance across healthcare facilities. Star ratings are also viewed favorably by consumers due to their simplicity and ease of interpretation. CMS developed its first "designation status" program in 2023 with the "Birth Friendly Designation" for hospitals that participate in quality improvement for maternal care.

Value-Based Purchasing Beyond Medicare

Medicaid, the state-based payer program, established quality reporting in the 2009 Children's Health Insurance Program (CHIP) Reauthorization Act. Medicaid maintains the Child, Adult, and Behavioral Health Core sets of measures, as well as a slate of measures for Home- and Community-Based Services. States have the option to report measures and may choose which measures to report although some reporting is now mandatory. CMMI also uses quality performance metrics within its multiple models. CMMI, established in 2010 as part of the ACA, seeks to identify innovative ways to improve healthcare quality and reduce costs. CMMI is committed to the Healthcare Payment Learning and Action Network (LAN) goal of moving 100% of traditional Medicare to value-based care through the adoption of two-sided risk alternative payment models. There have been over 40 various CMMI models to date. Some models have pioneered novel quality performance measures, such as the Social Drivers of Health (SDOH) screening measures and several patient-reported outcome measures, which have subsequently been adopted into Medicare FFS programs. Indeed, CMMI has an important role in the development of innovative quality performance measures. Some believe that true quality cannot be attained until payment models make this shift from volume-based payment to full value-based payment [7].

CMS Integrated System to Improve Quality

In addition to public reporting and quality measurement through VBPs, CMS has an interrelated system of payment, accountability, direct assistance, and auditing that supports a commitment to quality care. The CMS overarching framework of advancing quality is the CMS National Quality Strategy. Many areas across CMS work collaboratively to ensure alignment of strategies to improve quality and safety. CMS establishes baseline standards for safe, quality healthcare, helps foster a healthcare quality culture, provides direct quality improvement assistance, and determines coverage and payment. The Conditions of Participation set the minimum standards for quality and safety. Deeming organizations such as the Joint Commission and DNV GL Healthcare, as well as CMS directly, survey facilities to ensure these standards are met. Failure can result in a facility losing the ability to participate in Medicare and Medicaid. National quality improvement efforts, which provide technical assistance for achieving best outcomes are also supported through a broad network of Quality Improvement Organizations (QIO). The QIOs have focused on clinical outcomes, safety, equity, and interoperability with an emphasis of assisting nursing home facilities, small and rural hospitals, and small provider practices. The QIOs use additional quality measures across their programs.

Non-CMS Federal Roles for Quality Measurement

CMS is not the only federal agency to use quality performance measurement. The VHA and military health systems have a well-developed system of assessing quality performance and integrate many quality measures. Most recently, the VHA hospitals have begun reporting some of the traditional CMS quality measures. In 2023, the VHA participated for the first time in the Medicare Hospital Stars ratings program with favorable performance in quality metrics compared to non-VHA hospitals. The VHA also has a well organized, national system for safety reporting and improvement and is a leader in the use of High Reliability Organization (HRO) practices across its systems. HRO practices focus on minimizing errors and enhancing safety in complex, high-risk environments through a culture of mindfulness, accountability, and continuous learning. These practices emphasize five key principles: preoccupation with failure, reluctance to simplify interpretations, sensitivity to operations, commitment to resilience, and deference to expertise.

The CDC also develops and uses quality measurement, notably through their National Healthcare Safety Network (NHSN) for reporting of healthcare-acquired infections and other measures, especially for public health. During the COVID-19 pandemic, reporting to NHSN was greatly expanded to report national data on COVID cases, COVID vaccinations, and other data. As of 2024, NHSN has over 38,000 facilities, which participate in reporting data. In addition, CMS and CDC have further aligned around quality performance measurement, including joint initiatives on quality and safety measures such as a new Sepsis outcome measure.

AHRQ has long had a goal of promoting the highest quality and safety through research and education. AHRQ has played a pivotal role in measure development, including the patient experience measures (Consumer Assessment of Healthcare Providers & Systems [CAHPS] and Hospital CAHPS or HCAHPS) and the Patient Safety Indicator (PSI) measures. In addition, AHRQ maintains the national Patient Safety Organization data based – the Network of Patient Safety Databases, which aggregates non-identifiable national patient safety data. Other federal organizations also have established performance measurement programs, such as the HRSA Uniform Data System (UDS), in which federally qualified healthcare providers report on a core set of information, including health outcomes. HRSA also works closely with CMS to develop appropriate oversight of the organ transplant ecosystem. The Indian Health Services (IHS) hospitals generally follow the CMS Medicare FFS programs.

All combined, the federal government, through its multiple agencies and programs, its statutory authority for reporting and payment, and its QIO and VBP programs which integrate quality performance measurement, is a dominant driver for the use of quality measurement, and often "sets the bar" for what others follow.

Opportunities and Challenges of the Current Federal Value-Based Programs

Fragmentation

The evolution of multiple CMS VBPs, with different statutory authorities, designed and implemented at different times, with different policies and practices, has led to a somewhat fragmented approach to national quality accountability and transparency. Across these programs, numerous policies and practices are often not aligned. Rulemaking for these multiple programs occurs annually across multiple fiscal and calendar rules. Operational processes are different, including the audit processes, the policies for emergency circumstances and exceptions, the submission dates and frequencies, and the underlying information technology (IT) infrastructures of each program. This may lead to confusion, especially for large healthcare systems that report to multiple programs. Though there have been proposals aimed at greater alignment across programs, Congressional action is required for significant change.

Burden

Providers have voiced concerns about the burden of reporting to these programs and about the lack of alignment of quality measures [8]. Consumers are often confused about the multiple metrics reported across programs. However, it is not just the "burden" of CMS programs; many organizations find their "burden" compounded by other quality measurement programs. Commercial payer quality reporting and payment programs are also each different and often change with every contract. Specialty societies and clinical registries may also utilize other measures that may not align. For example, the definitions of hypertension or diabetes quality may be different across different programs. Multiple quality improvement programs may utilize additional and non-aligned metrics. Other regulators and accrediting agencies, such as the Joint Commission and the National Committee for Quality Assurance (NCQA), utilize other different measures and programs. And finally, multiple rating agencies use yet more [9]. A facility or healthcare system may need a dedicated team just to keep abreast of all the changing requirements and reporting mandates.

Adequacy of Incentive/Penalty

The penalties and incentives are variable and relatively modest. Nearly half the CMS VBP are pay for reporting only – meaning organizations must report data or face a penalty (generally 2% of Annual Payment Update [APU]), however actual performance does not impact payment. The other programs, which are pay for performance, have variable incentives and penalties ranging from the HVBP, which, as a net neutral program can provide incentives based on the penalties accrued, to the HRRP, which is largely a penalty program of up to 3% of Medicare payments. The clinician program MIPS has the largest potential maximal positive and negative adjustments of 9%. Some operational and financial officers have chosen to accept penalties rather than fix underlying issues. Nonetheless, despite the challenges of public and private VBPs, these value-based efforts have indeed promoted change and improvements in quality and safety. These payment and public reporting programs (combined with other quality improvement efforts such as QIOs) have arguably led to additional quality focus by healthcare leaders and governance boards, the establishment of quality, safety, and experience departments, the expansion of analytics, which support quality improvement, data, and electronic medical record systems, which support quality improvement, and the establishment of learning healthcare facilities and systems that engage in ongoing efforts for continuous improvement. Indeed, reports do indicate an improvement in overall healthcare quality. The 2019 National Healthcare Quality and Disparities Report from AHRQ noted that the quality of healthcare improved generally through 2018, but the pace of improvement varied by priority area. Recent CMS data shows that pre-pandemic, 88% of analyzed measures had improved or stable performance [10]. However, during the COVID pandemic, over 50% of measures exhibited worse than expected results. Are these efforts of quality measurement integrated into payment VBP enough to make significant change? It is unclear – but without these programs, it is possible the focus on quality would be lessened or lost.

Integration of Quality Measures in CMS Value-Based Programs and Public Reporting: Measure Development, Inclusion, and Removal

The expansion of the multiple CMS VBPs was met with an expansion of quality measures and measurement tools, including measures development, measures management systems, and processes for review, endorsement, maintenance, and inclusion and exclusion of measures into these programs. As of 2024, CMS uses 492 unique active measures across 26 programs. This is a notable decrease from the past inventory from 764 in 2017, due to Meaningful Measures (described below) and efforts to remove duplication and retire weaker measures. A large proportion of measures are in the MIPS program (201 MIPS measures; not inclusive of qualified clinical data registry [QCDR]/other registry measures). This is because of the statutory requirements of MIPS to have quality performance measures for all specialties and cost measures to account for 50% of Medicare Part A (hospital) and Part B (physician) spending. CMS stewards about a third of the measures used in their programs, with NCQA being the next most common measure steward. This is followed by various other organizations, including the CDC, AHRQ, Pharmacy Quality Alliance, and several specialty society organizations. Of the three types of measures in the Donabedian framework (outcome, process, and structure), CMS VBP utilizes 251 process measures, 204 outcome measures, 8 structural measures, and 29 cost measures. The proportion of outcome measures continues to increase. Each type of measure has its own advantages and disadvantages. In addition, there has been an intentional shift to measures that are digitally sourced, with nearly 90% of measures on the 2024 current measures under consideration (MUC) list meeting this definition. More and more electronic clinical quality measures (eCQMs) have been introduced over time, with 67 eCQM in place in 2024.

Strategic Priorities for the Development of Quality Measures for CMS Value-Based Programs: Quality Frameworks

There have been several strategic frameworks to guide the prioritization, development, and use of quality measures in CMS VBP. In March 2011, the first National Quality Strategy was established to improve the delivery of healthcare services, patient health outcomes, and population health as a nationwide effort to improve health and healthcare across America. It was designed by public and private stakeholders to provide an opportunity to align quality measures and quality improvement activities. Its aims were "Better Health, Better Care, Lower Costs," and it aligned with the Institute for Healthcare Improvement (IHI) Triple Aims of that time (improving the patient experience of care, improving the health of populations, and reducing the per capita cost of healthcare). This strategy included multiple federal agencies, including CMS, CDC, AHRQ, HRSA, Administration for Community Living (ACL), Office of Personnel Management (OPM), and Substance Abuse and Mental Health Services Administration (SAMHSA). Other non-government initiatives aligned with this strategy, including Blue Cross Blue Shield of Massachusetts, the California Department of Healthcare Services, and several children's hospitals and programs. This was followed by a flurry of other quality strategies, including Million Hearts (CDC), the CMS quality strategy (2013), and the then 11th Statement of work from the QIO network (2014).

In 2016, CMS began its work on the Meaningful Measures Framework for quality measurement to continue the strategic prioritization and selection of quality measurement used in its programs. Meaningful Measures 1.0 outlined a set of 6 priority areas and 19 goals. Over the next several years, the number of measures used across the CMS VBP was reduced in line with the focused priorities and as a commitment to reducing provider/facility burden from measurement, as noted earlier. The Meaningful Measures Framework continued to evolve to MM 2.0 in 2021, with 8 standalone priority areas. During this time, HHS also released its National Health Quality Roadmap (May 2020), which called for a strategy for establishing, adopting, and publishing common quality measures; aligning inpatient and outpatient measures; and the elimination of low-value or counterproductive measures. The plan sought a significant reduction in measure burden and to reform how measures are used in federal programs.

In 2022, CMS released its new CMS National Quality Strategy, with input from a wide array of stakeholders. The CMS National Quality Strategy is an aligned cross-cutting initiative (CCI) across the Agency (1 of 13 CCI). It is an ongoing, ever-evolving strategy. It prioritizes eight focus areas for quality, some of which are new or evolved from prior national strategies, to include an expanded focus on equity, safety, innovation, resilience, patient/individual engagement, and scientific innovation. In addition, the CMS National Quality strategy, includes a focus on outcomes, with a special focus on certain areas such as maternal health and safety, behavioral health and substance use disorders, diabetes, HIV/AIDS, and cancer. Finally, the strategy places an emphasis on alignment of quality strategies, measures, and programs across CMS and, to the degree feasible, across federal, state, and private sectors.

These multiple frameworks have guided measures prioritized for development and subsequent use in CMS programs. Through annual rulemaking, CMS shapes the VBPs through measures to meet these goals.

Federal Processes and Reports to Support Measures Development and Use

In addition to developing quality measures following the goals and priorities of the CMS National Quality Strategy, CMS maintains extensive measures support tools called the Measures Management System. This includes the CMS Measures Inventory Tool (CMIT), the Measures Under Consideration Entry and Review Information Tool (MERIT), publication of the annual Measures Under Consideration list (MUC), the digital eCQI resource center, the Measures Blueprint (a "gold standard" book on measures development), the Quality Measure Index (QMI) for measure evaluation/scoring, and the Measure Authoring Development Integrated Environment (MADIE) tool for eCQMs testing.

CMS produces reports regarding measure development and progress as mandated by SSA 1890/1890A. CMS produces an annual Report to Congress (RTC) on quality measurement. The latest Report to Congress – "Identification of Quality Measurement Priorities: Strategic Plan, Initiatives, and Activities" was published in December 2023 and discusses the strategies and priorities, as well as funding for quality measurement. CMS is prioritizing the development and use of digital measures and focusing efforts in addressing health inequities, patient-reported outcomes, and rural health concerns [11].

Additionally, CMS produces triennial reports to Congress on the National Impact Assessment of Quality Measures as required by SSA 1890A(a) [12], intended to help the public and Federal Government understand the impact of

CMS's quality measurement investments and consider future needs. The latest report was released in February 2024 and analyzed quality measure results from 2016 to 2021. Findings show that improvements in measure performance, largely prior to the COVID pandemic, were associated with positive impacts for millions of patients and substantial costs avoided. Performance fell during the COVID pandemic, although newer reports, suggest that quality performance is once again improving.

Measure development, as outlined throughout this book, is a multi-year strategic commitment. From conceptualization to the determination of measure specification, to testing, to proposing for use in a CMS VBP generally takes from two to four years, with an average cost of approximately $750,000 USD per measure. Any individual or organization can submit a measure to be considered by CMS for use in its VBP through the MERIT system for the MUC list. Should a measure be favorably reviewed, it may be proposed for rulemaking (generally the following year), which, if finalized, would be implemented in yet a subsequent year. The entire time from conceptualization to inclusion of a quality measure in a CMS VBP is, on average, five years.

Opportunities and Challenges of Quality Measurement in CMS Value-Based Programs

Such an extensive, complicated quality measurement ecosystem creates both opportunities and challenges.

Alignment/Lack of Alignment

Given the multiple VBPs that utilize measures, each with their own policies, combined with multiple measures to cover all facility types and specialties, it is unsurprising that quality measures are not always aligned. A healthcare system may have to report similar but not identical measures (e.g., different versions of measures for blood pressure control or diabetes control). The lack of a true National Quality Measurement Strategy underpins some of the challenge of alignment.

Multiple attempts have been and continue to be made to better align quality measurement across all CMS (and external) programs. This includes the cross-CMS quality workgroup, which has been working to align measures across Medicare FFS, MA, Medicaid and CHIP, CMMI, and Marketplace. In 2023, CMS published its "Universal Foundation" of measures, beginning with a set of ambulatory adult and pediatric measures, in an effort to standardize across CMS (and external), the measures that are of highest priority and specify which measure(s) to use both in and across programs [13].

In future iterations, CMS plans to add to the Universal Foundation, in a building-block manner, such as a hospital set of measures, post-acute care, and specific disease-specific sets (such as maternal health). Finally, CMS is aligning ambulatory specialty measures through the transition of the MIPS program to the MIPS Value Pathway (MVP) program. Whereas the MIPS program offers clinicians a wide choice of over 200 measures for reporting, the MVP program creates "sub-groups," or sets of aligned, cohesive quality measures with associated and aligned cost measures, improvement activities, and promotion of interoperability. CMS plans for the MVP to represent the aligned "Universal Foundation" of measures for specific specialties or conditions, while at the same time reducing confusion and burden and ensuring measures that are meaningful to clinicians and patients.

CMS is also spearheading efforts at aligning measures across Federal partners, including CDC, AHRQ, HRSA, VHA, National Institutes of Health (NIH), and others. Recently CMS has initiated cross-agency reviews of the MUC, as well as other measure alignment strategies, to create better efficiency, reduce duplication of efforts across agencies, and use a single set of quality performance measures across all Federal agencies to the degree feasible. More and more, CMS is working collaboratively on measure development such as the new sepsis outcome measure with CDC, revised patient experience measures with AHRQ, behavioral health integration measures with AHRQ and SAMHSA, and safety measures across the HHS Leadership Alliance for Safety with AHRQ, CDC, CMS, and FDA.

Finally, there are attempts at alignment across all payers, most notably the Core Quality Measurement Collaborative (CQMC), co-led by America's Health Insurance Plans (AHIP), CMS, and the CBE. To date, CQMC has identified 10 core sets of ambulatory measure sets that it hopes will serve as the standard for use in these areas. In addition, the CQMC has been addressing a standard approach to digital measurement and a standard approach to patient-reported outcome measures.

Burden of Measurement Reporting

There have been numerous concerns voiced on the burden of reporting quality measures [14, 15]. Within CMS, the Office of Healthcare Experience and Interoperability (OHEI) has led efforts on human-centered design and stakeholder engagement on how to reduce burden. Quality measurement reporting was high on the list of burdens, although not the highest burden. As noted earlier, this led to attempts to streamline measures across CMS through the Meaningful Measures initiative, as well as the ongoing efforts at alignment. To the degree feasible, CMS has made efforts to retire measures according to the measure removal criteria set forward in policy and to remove measures from programs whenever new measures are proposed to be added.

The burden of measurement reporting, however, is not just due to numbers; it is also dependent on the measure type and collection methodology. In the past, the widespread use of claims measures was a way to reduce burden. However, claims reporting fails to capture rich clinical information available in electronic medical records. A recent paper from Johns Hopkins University outlines the cost and efforts of measures' collection and reporting. It demonstrated that claims based and chart-abstracted measures are the most burdensome and costly to report, whereas digital measures (eCQMs), once built, are much less expensive and burdensome [16]. They reported that the average claims-based measure cost $37,553 per measure/year, while the cost for electronic measures was $1,901 per measure/year. Finally, continued advances for alignment and standardization of measures will help relieve the burden.

Managing to the Measures

Does the measurement framework and utilization in multiple CMS VBP lead to providers/facilities only "managing to the test" and not devoting resources to other quality improvements that may not be part of the "list" of measures? Do providers/facilities "game" the system to look better on a dashboard? It is difficult to answer these questions, although anecdotes abound, which suggest that both are true. In the end, the pursuit of the highest quality and safest care must be an organizational culture and commitment with ongoing, perpetual, everlasting efforts embedded within every organization to create continuous excellence through a learning health system.

Confusion and Lack of Understanding of Measurement Data

Through the many VBP and quality improvement programs, both government and commercial, providers, payers, and facilities have become much more aware of the expectations for quality improvement and have developed an understanding of the measures, although detailed understanding is sometimes problematic. Many efforts have been taken to ensure that public measurement information is comprehensive, comprehensible, and directed to topics of interest to stakeholders. The Stars ratings systems, for example, are a way of combining multiple measures into a single rating for ease of understanding large amounts of data. Yet, just reviewing the overall Star rating in many of the CMS programs may not provide the total picture of what is happening in a facility and may also represent a time delay with respect to recent events. For example, icons to demonstrate a history of abuse have recently been added to the Nursing Home Compare program to provide clear information on factors, which are important to residents and families. With the rise of consumerism, education, and outreach and engagement programs, consumers are becoming more and more savvy about these measures and are beginning to use these tools to make healthcare choices. Perhaps more important, payers often use the measures and CMS VBP to make assessments about providers to include in networks and provider groups. For example, accountable care organizations may also utilize this data in making choices about who to include in those networks.

Attribution

Is the measure, or the program, directly attributable to the facility or individual clinician? These are questions frequently raised, which is why testing of measures at the level in which the measure is intended for use is important [17]. Specific challenges arise with small facilities or individual/small practices, where relatively small numbers of patients can reduce the reliability of measurement. Most measures mandate a certain volume of data submission to be included to counteract low-volume concerns. In addition, whether a specific provider is included or excluded in a measure, as defined in the measure specifications, is often a topic of debate. This has been particularly true of the MIPS cost measures, where attributing cost to a specific provider requires detailed measure inclusion/exclusion criteria. Measurement development utilizes Technical Expert Panels representing multiple diverse backgrounds to review the evidence and help make these complex decisions of attribution.

Risk Adjustment

Within any given program, do comparisons of facilities/providers "fairly" account for different patient and population characteristics? There is a great deal of attention to risk adjustment models in the CMS VBP. Most measures are risk adjusted for clinical differences.

Validity

The development process of measures includes extensive testing for feasibility, validity, and reliability and assessing for potential unintended consequences. However, are the auditing programs and data validation processes robust enough to identify issues of gaming, or false submission, or accidental error? A review process is embedded into each VBP whereby facilities/clinicians receive preview data and have an opportunity to look for error. However, the overall audit process for the measures is limited.

Future Strategies for Integration of Quality Measurement in Federal Value-Based Programs

The evaluation of quality, experience, safety, access, and cost will remain a foundation for determining "value" in healthcare. America still spends more than any country for healthcare, and yet has some of the lowest-performing quality metrics [18]. Until this course is reversed, ongoing efforts will seek to advance this. Future changes in payment, quality measures, data strategies, and learning systems offer potential paths to improvement.

Interoperable Digital Data

Perhaps the most important alignment and burden reduction strategy, and data robustness improvement, is the transition of quality measures to using digital data with standardized definitions and data elements, with reporting via Fast Healthcare Interoperability Resources (FHIR/FHIR APIs). Digital data can provide seamless and real-time (or near real time) reporting. CMS has committed to fully digital quality measurement in its FFS VBP. While the time frame remains a challenge, significant efforts are already underway. In 2024, almost 90% of measures under consideration were digitally sourced. NCQA is also moving toward digital measures. CMS collaborates closely with the Assistant Secretary for Technology Policy (ASTP) on promoting interoperability, including through the Promoting Interoperability VBP for hospitals and clinicians and the standardization of data elements through the United States Core Data Information (USCDI) set and USCDI+. The aspiration is for a fully integrated, interoperable, digital data system where quality measures are a byproduct of the clinical workflow and not a burden to providers; where these data can be utilized in real time for clinical decision support, and where data supports an ongoing learning health system for continuous improvement. Additionally, a digital quality measurement structure allows for the benefit of layering on advanced analytics such as predictive analysis and AI tools.

Advanced Analytics/Machine Learning and Artificial Intelligence (AI)

The year 2024 is an inflection point for AI, which could transform quality measurement into new directions. However, asking AI to "find the best quality hospital for hip replacement surgery" will still rely on the defined data collection systems and algorithms to answer such questions. It becomes even more essential that the data in these measures is accurate, unbiased, reliable, valid, and tested. The algorithms behind these advanced analytics also need to be accurate, unbiased, reliable, valid, and tested, and end users must be aware of potential issues and unintended consequences. President Biden released an Executive Order in 2023 to require HHS and other federal departments to develop a plan to reflect these goals.

New Areas of Focus for Quality Measurement in VBP

Newer opportunities for quality and safety performance measures within CMS VBP will emerge. Expanded Patient Reporting Outcomes Measures (PROM) is a key commitment of the CMS National Quality Strategy. CMS is developing a framework for new PROMs and collaborating with AHRQ on revisions to current patient experience metrics. New areas of focus for safety include diagnostic excellence, safety of the electronic medical record (and AI systems), and more robust, real-time harm reporting. New efforts will be developed for clinical outcomes, including prevention, well-being and reduction of chronic disease burden.

Payment Systems

It is unclear if systems to ensure highest quality, safety, access, and experience can be fully implemented in a fee for service payment environment. Aggressive movement toward two-sided, advanced risk arrangements, with inherent additional flexibility to provide non-traditional services, is already underway, led by innovation models, Medicare Advantage, and ACO programs. Some programs have shown trends toward higher quality care at lower cost. However, not all models have demonstrated significant quality improvement. It is not yet entirely clear if this transition is able to achieve the quality goals and bend the cost curve. However, continued models, continued transformation, and continued commitment to change will help evolve the healthcare ecosystem to one of greater value. New payment programs will need innovative quality measures that focus on impactful outcomes from a population viewpoint.

Summary: The Role of Government in Quality Measurement Integration

The Federal government has a pivotal role in advancing the use of quality performance measurement to ensure accountability, transparency, and public information and to drive improvements for quality, safety, access, experience, and cost. Quality reporting is now a core function in healthcare, as it enables value-based payments, provider comparisons, and consumer choice. Although there are inherent challenges, especially within a complex and fragmented healthcare system, in general, care and outcomes have improved through these efforts. Yet, the COVID-19 pandemic also reminded us that quality infrastructures and systems are not always resilient. Ensuring high-quality care requires ongoing support and "hard wiring" into all healthcare practices, within a learning health system committed to ongoing improvement and a dedication to the best care for all individuals.

Discussion Questions

11.1 How has the US Federal Government, particularly CMS, shaped the integration of quality performance measurement into VBPs?

11.2 What level of incentives, including potential penalties in VBPs, will likely drive significant changes in provider behavior? What alternative strategies might be more effective?

11.3 Given the concerns raised about the burden of reporting for quality measures, what solutions could be implemented to streamline reporting while maintaining accuracy and comprehensiveness?

11.4 How effective are current strategies, such as stratifying quality measures by race, ethnicity, and dual eligibility, in addressing healthcare inequities? What additional strategies could be taken to ensure equitable care?

11.5 With the emergence of digital data, AI, and patient-reported outcome measures (PROMs), what potential transformations do you foresee in quality measurement systems? How can these technologies address current limitations and challenges?

Note: The views expressed in this chapter are those of the authors and do not necessarily reflect the official policy or position of the United States government or any agency thereof. The opinions expressed here do not represent the official opinions of a specific federal agency.

References

1 Fiore, J.A., Madison, A.J., Poisal, J.A. et al. (2024). National health expenditure projections, 2023-32: payer trends diverge as pandemic-related policies fade. *Health Aff. (Millwood)* 43 (7): 910–921. https://doi.org/10.1377/hlthaff.2024.00469.

2 La Rochelle, P. and Julien, A.S. (2013). How dramatic were the effects of handwashing on maternal mortality observed by Ignaz Semmelweis? *J. R. Soc. Med.* 106 (11): 459–460. https://doi.org/10.1177/0141076813507843.

3 Nightingale, F. (1863). *Notes on Hospitals*, 3e. Longman, Green, Longman, Roberts and Green.

4 Codman, E.A. (1918). *A Study in Hospital Efficiency: As Demonstrated by the Case Report of the First Five Years of a Private Hospital.* Thomas Todd.

5 Davey, P., Thakore, S., and Tully, V. (2022). How to embed quality improvement into medical training. *BMJ* 376: e055084. https://doi.org/10.1136/bmj-2020-055084.

6 Bond, A.M., Schpero, W.L., Casalino, L.P. et al. (2022). Association between individual primary care physician merit-based incentive payment system score and measures of process and patient outcomes. *JAMA* 328 (21): 2136–2146. https://doi.org/10.1001/jama.2022.20619.

7 Shenfeld, D.K., Navathe, A.S., and Emanuel, E.J. (2024). The promise and challenge of value-based payment. *JAMA Intern. Med.* 184 (7): 716–717. https://doi.org/10.1001/jamainternmed.2024.1343.

8 Khullar, D., Bond, A.M., O'Donnell, E.M. et al. (2021). Time and financial costs for physician practices to participate in the Medicare merit-based incentive payment system: a qualitative study. *JAMA Health Forum* 2 (5): e210527. https://doi.org/10.1001/jamahealthforum.2021.0527.

9 Bilimoria, K.Y., Birkmeyer, J.D., and Burstin, H. (2019). Rating the raters: an evaluation of publicly reported hospital quality rating systems. *NEJM Catal.* 5 (4). https://doi.org/10.1056/CAT.19.0629.

10 Fleisher, L.A., Schreiber, M., Cardo, D., and Srinivasan, A. (2022). Health care safety during the pandemic and beyond – building a system that ensures resilience. *N. Eng. J. Med.* 386 (7): 609–611. https://doi.org/10.1056/NEJMp2118285.

11 CMS (2023). 2023 report to congress – identification of quality measurement priorities: strategic plan, initiatives, and activities (PDF). https://www.cms.gov/files/document/fy20231890rtcfinalpdf.pdf.

12 Jacobs, D., Rawal, P., Schreiber, M. et al. (2024). Update on the Medicare value-based care strategy: alignment, growth, equity. https://www.healthaffairs.org/content/forefront/update-medicare-value-based-care-strategy-alignment-growth-equity.

13 Jacobs, D.B., Schreiber, M., Seshamani, M. et al. (2023). Aligning quality measures across CMS – The Universal Foundation. *N. Eng. J. Med.* 388 (9): 776–779. https://doi.org/10.1056/NEJMp2215539.

14 Gettel, C.J., Suter, L.G., Bagshaw, K. et al. (2024). Patient-reported outcome-based performance measures in alternative payment models: current use, implementation barriers, and principles to succeed. *Value Health* 27 (2): 199–205. https://doi.org/10.1016/j.jval.2023.10.017.

15 Husaini, M. and Joynt Maddox, K.E. (2020). Paying for performance improvement in quality and outcomes of cardiovascular care: challenges and prospects. *Methodist Debakey Cardiovasc. J.* 16 (3): 225–231. https://doi.org/10.14797/mdcj-16-3-225.

16 Saraswathula, A., Merck, S.J., Bai, G. et al. (2023). The volume and cost of quality metric reporting. *JAMA* 329 (21): 1840–1847. https://doi.org/10.1001/jama.2023.7271.

17 Riley, W., Love, K., and Wilson, C. (2023). Patient attribution-A call for a system redesign. *JAMA Health Forum* 4 (3): e225527. https://doi.org/10.1001/jamahealthforum.2022.5527.

18 Gunja, M.Z., Gumas, E.D., and Williams, R.D. (2023). U.S. Health Care from a global perspective, 2022: accelerating spending, worsening outcomes. https://www.commonwealthfund.org/publications/issue-briefs/2023/jan/us-health-care-global-perspective-2022.

12 Improving Diagnostic Safety and Quality in Healthcare Through Measurement

Karen S. Cosby

Department of Emergency Medicine, Rush University Medical Center and Attending Physician, Cook County Health, Chicago, IL, USA

Quality measurement is firmly embedded in the US healthcare system. Participation in quality programs is required for accreditation and payment. Some are critical of the enormous investment in what has been referred to as an overly expansive "quality measurement enterprise" that has generated thousands of quality measures that cost healthcare systems millions of dollars per year [1]. Despite the abundance of measures, relatively few clinical quality measures focus on diagnostic quality and safety. The lack of attention to diagnostic quality may be due to a variety of reasons: diagnostic performance has historically been considered the purview of clinicians and the responsibility of educators, medical boards, and licensing agencies; labels of diagnostic error sometimes seem subjective, or cases too complex, or too difficult to standardize or measure; and lastly, there has been a lack of awareness of the extent of diagnostic safety events and the harm they cause. That is beginning to change.

Importance of Diagnostic Safety Measurement

Diagnostic errors are now recognized as significant, harmful, and pervasive throughout all healthcare settings. In 2015, the National Academies (NA) declared improving diagnosis to be a "moral, professional, and public health imperative" [2].

Quality Measurement in Healthcare, First Edition. Edited by Jesse M. Pines, Helen Burstin, and Jane Hyatt Thorpe.
© 2025 Jesse M. Pines, Helen Burstin, and Jane Hyatt Thorpe.
Published 2025 by John Wiley & Sons Ltd.

An accurate and timely diagnosis is essential to determine what interventions can optimize patient outcome. A wrong, missed, or delayed diagnosis allows the healthcare problem(s) to persist and even worsen; a wrong label or misdiagnosis can lead to unnecessary medical interventions and treatments that add risk without potential benefit.

Leading studies on the incidence of diagnostic errors note the following:

- Diagnostic errors are among the most common causes of preventable medical errors [3].
- Studies from closed, paid malpractice claims identify diagnostic errors as a leading source of harm (accounting for 23–28.6% of all claims). Diagnosis-related claims generate the highest payouts [4, 5].
- Compared with other claims, diagnosis-related claims result in greater disability and are more than twice as likely to result in death [5].
- Diagnostic errors occur in 5.08% of outpatient visits, affecting 12 million adults each year, half of whom likely experience severe harm [6].
- Diagnostic errors have been identified in 5.6% of patients requiring readmission within 7 days of hospital discharge [7].
- Each of us may likely experience a diagnostic error during our lifetime [6].

Despite considerable focus on improving patient safety, progress in diagnostic safety has lagged considerably behind other efforts. Some lament that "diagnostic errors don't get any respect" and are "neglected" [8, 9]. If we are to address diagnostic error, we need methods to identify and learn from them, the ability to mitigate harm, and preferably, strategies to improve. Measurement is integral to improvement.

Foundational Definitions and a Unifying Framework for Diagnosis

Measurement begins with defining terms and specifications, and for that, we need agreement for basic definitions.

A diagnosis is the label we give that best explains the patient's healthcare problem that is premised on the best current scientific understanding of pathophysiology. Diagnostic errors usually refer to a wrong label applied to a condition or a flaw in the process of diagnosis that leads to a delayed or wrong diagnosis.

In 2015, the NA produced a breakthrough report, *Improving Diagnosis in Healthcare*, that provides a unifying framework for conceptualizing the diagnostic process [2]. That authoritative work provides a definition for diagnostic error and describes a framework that provides useful targets for measurement and improvement efforts.

The NA expert working group defined diagnostic error as:

> *the failure to (a) establish an accurate and timely explanation of the patient's health problem(s) or (b) communicate that explanation to the patient.*

The NA framework, shown in Figure 12.1 and detailed in their report, describes the diagnostic journey patients experience using a sociotechnical model that views diagnosis as an iterative process occurring over a variable time period, involving engagement of the patient with clinicians, consultants, and other team members, sometimes across multiple healthcare settings and sites. The report acknowledges that diagnostic problems may be complex, and in some cases, their pathways highly variable as the work progresses in the face of uncertainty. The model includes the entire trajectory of the patient through the healthcare system back to home and community and acknowledges the multiple interactions between patients and clinicians within a complicated network of loosely integrated processes. The authors emphasized that diagnostic problems should be approached from a systems perspective to improve infrastructure supportive of optimal processes, and it placed responsibility for diagnostic quality on healthcare organizations.

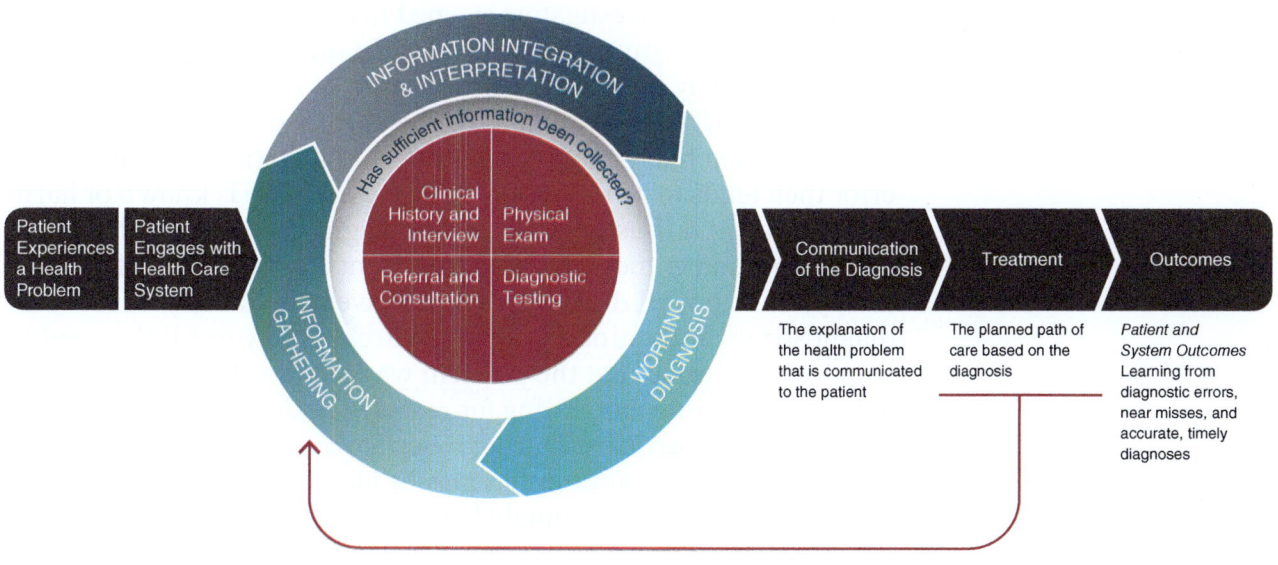

TIME

Figure 12.1: National academies framework for diagnosis.

Source: Reproduced from Ref. [2] / National Academy of Sciences.

Conceptual Approaches to Defining and Measuring Diagnostic Failure

Researchers and those engaged in quality improvement have used a variety of approaches for measurement of diagnostic failure. Six models currently dominate the field and influence what types of methods are used to identify and measure diagnostic quality, and each provides differing strategies for improvement (Table 12.1).

1. **Traditional clinician-centric approach:** A historical model views diagnosis as a cognitive process. This view holds individual clinicians accountable for their diagnostic outcomes and errors. Professionals address diagnostic failures through education and training, self-reflection, efforts to obtain feedback on their performance and their patient outcomes, and increased exposure and experience with clinical cases through case reviews and simulations. Individuals are usually responsible for tracking and learning from their errors on their own. And while individual expertise is necessary, even the most expert clinicians cannot assure quality care absent a supportive system. There are no standard approaches to measurement of individual clinicians' diagnostic performance.

2. **Diagnostic error:** The patient safety literature defines error as the use of a wrong plan to achieve an aim or failure to complete the plan as intended [10, 11]. Investigators steeped in patient safety have defined diagnosis error as any mistake or failure in the diagnostic process that results in a delay in diagnosis or a missed or misdiagnosis [12]. The concept of diagnostic error came to be used to describe any suboptimal action that likely contributed to a poor outcome. The judgment of error then tends to be made only after the outcome is known or harm is identified and thus is subject to hindsight and outcome bias. The definition is sometimes applied independent of assessments of preventability; thus, not all diagnostic errors have actionability. A focus on diagnostic error dominated early research largely to fill the need to convincingly argue that the problem was relevant for the population at large and to impact funding for research and public policy.

3. **Missed opportunities:** During investigations of delayed or missed diagnoses, missed opportunities may be identified that, had they been recognized or acted upon, might have yielded better outcomes. Certain patterns of these opportunities have been used to detect common system problems that create risk. This concept has been applied retroactively, after harm is identified, but has also been applied prospectively to detect opportunities to rescue before irreversible harm occurs. (See the trigger method below.) This categorization provides a dimension of preventability and actionability to the label of an error.

Table 12.1: Conceptual approaches to defining and measuring diagnostic quality and safety.

Foundational definition	Data source for measurement	Measurement method	Improvement strategy	Authority
Diagnosis: focus on cognition and clinician/team performance	Quality not typically tracked proactively "Interesting" or select cases may be identified through random discovery or referral by individuals Review of EHRs and clinical records	Routine diagnostic quality is not measured by most centers	Focuses on individuals: ▪ Education ▪ Improving feedback ▪ Simulation ▪ Teamwork training	Licensing boards Professional organizations
Diagnostic error: focus on failure	Retrospective reviews of events: ▪ Autopsy data ▪ Malpractice claims ▪ Patient complaints ▪ Investigation of sentinel and adverse events or unexpected outcomes ▪ Error reporting systems	Event-centric and reactive as cases are identified Some may use dashboard to record high risk cases SPADE (look-back and look-forward to identify missed cases)	Error avoidance Surveillance of similar cases Discussion at academic conferences, such as Mortality and Morbidity reviews	Local institution Public health or regulatory bodies may investigate if reported
Missed opportunities: focus on compliance with expected guidelines or recommended actions	Prospective design of health system informatics Relies on EHR	Triggers	Specific resources designed to match to individual triggers	Local, regional health system
Diagnostic safety, diagnostic adverse events	Investigation of event reports or referrals related to harm or monitoring programs Can be designed by QI programs	Convenient sample based on referring source Cases with harm may be identified by: ▪ Incidental discovery ▪ Risk Manager review ▪ Peer Review ▪ Malpractice claim ▪ Formal report system ▪ Trigger	System designed to mitigate or minimize risk	Health system or regulator

(Continued)

Table 12.1: (Continued)

Foundational definition	Data source for measurement	Measurement method	Improvement strategy	Authority
Diagnostic quality, diagnostic excellence	Prospective Informatics support for specific processes	Supported by quality measures	New policies and processes Systems engineering System design	Can be regulated by local, state, national authorities and lead to guidelines and policies
Patient experience	Patient complaints Patient surveys Patient interviews	Depending on method, reports may be spontaneous or solicited	May provide ideas for local QI activities	Local or regional health-care systems; participation may be required for national systems such as Press Gainey or HCAHPS (although they currently lack specific diagnosis related themes)

Abbreviations: EHR, electronic health record; SPADE, symptom–disease pair analysis of diagnostic error; QI, quality improvement; HCAHPS, hospital consumer assessment of healthcare providers and systems.

4. **Diagnostic safety events, diagnostic adverse events, and undesirable diagnostic events** focus on harm that patients experience when their diagnosis is wrong or delayed. Most commonly, these approaches focus on the identification of errors in event reporting, although some apply it to the proactive identification of high-risk conditions and settings that are most likely to suffer adverse outcomes [13].

5. **Diagnostic excellence and diagnostic quality:** These terms draw from the quality paradigm that focuses on achieving quality (not just avoiding error) that includes an optimal process that is accurate, timely, cost-effective, safe, patient-centric, and equitable [14]. A focus on measurement for diagnostic quality defines specific goals or standards for clinical problems.

6. **Patient experience and outcomes:** Much of traditional quality improvement views quality from the perspective of clinicians. But ultimately, what matters most is how patients assess the quality of their care. Patients have the most to gain by optimizing their care and, as the only constant throughout their diagnostic trajectory, they have a deep understanding of the entirety of the diagnostic process. Patient interviews and surveys reveal that they can add substantively to our understanding of diagnostic quality [15].

Methods of Measuring Diagnostic Quality and Safety

A variety of methods have been used to identify and measure diagnostic quality. The major features that distinguish the methods relate to their underlying conceptual framework (described above), the purpose of measurement, whether or not the method is retrospective or prospective, and how they relate to improvement strategies.

Symptom-Disease Pair Analysis of Diagnostic Error (SPADE)

From an institutional and even health policy perspective, it is meaningful to benchmark diagnostic performance for certain common or risk-prone diagnoses. One approach has been developed that pairs specific conditions to one or more common symptoms to detect diagnostic errors that had prior visits that failed to recognize either the disease or risk of progression to a more serious problem. Using a longitudinal database that captures care within a given system, the Symptom-Disease Pair Analysis of Diagnostic Error (SPADE) methodology looks back from the time of an index diagnosis (e.g., acute myocardial infarction [MI]) to determine if a related symptom (e.g., chest pain) was present at a prior visit and if so, may have predicted potential harm to come that might have been preventable [16]. From a general database of visits, other cases with that symptom are then used to look forward to see if the index diagnosis occurs at a rate beyond what is expected from other conditions that might prompt a repeat medical evaluation. If so, the symptom-disease pair is validated. This "look back, look forward" method requires a longitudinal database to benchmark the frequency of specific missed diagnoses. It may prove useful for population estimates of harm to help institutions track their performance against intra- or inter-institutional performance. The SPADE methodology has been used to establish error rates for appendicitis [17], stroke [18], MI [19], and sepsis [20].

There are a number of limitations of the technique. It requires a large longitudinal data set and, for uncommon events, a long evaluation period [21]. The symptom-disease pairing will miss cases in which the primary diagnostic code differs even slightly from the defined symptom – including atypical or complex cases. The use of administrative data lacks granularity to provide context for the miss and thus, opportunity to determine if the miss was preventable given available knowledge and circumstances at the time. Since it is retrospective, it is not useful to intervene on any specific case. However, the method represents an advancement in measuring the incidence of specific patterns of missed or delayed diagnoses and can provide evidence for potential gaps in quality that need attention.

Error Reporting Systems

Robust error reporting systems have been credited with safety improvement in other industries, but development and uptake of error reporting have been slow in healthcare. Routine manual or electronic reporting systems for diagnostic adverse events and safety problems are in their infancy. The Agency for Healthcare Research and Quality (AHRQ) recently released a guide for common formats to standardize event reporting for diagnostic errors, but it has not yet been widely implemented [22]. Error reports can uncover particularly consequential patterns of error but are unlikely to provide reliable measurement for frequency of events. In fact, there may be an inverse relationship between the number of reports and the frequency of events, since an increase in reports may well reflect improvement in culture and transparency that are the mark of a learning health system.

Electronic Surveillance and Trigger Tools

More success has been had with trigger tools designed to capture potential safety events. The Institute for Healthcare Improvement (IHI) global trigger tool provides a list of events that may signal an adverse event that can be detected in a brief record review [23]. It largely focuses on medication and operative complications, but recent work has identified potential triggers for diagnostic adverse events. Examples of targets for diagnostic trigger tools include an unexpected return to hospital after a discharge, an unusual length of stay for a given diagnosis, unexpected escalation of care or transfer to a higher level of care, and failure to follow up after abnormal test results. Triggers have been developed for a variety of problems and settings, including pediatrics [24], oncology [25], intensive care units [26], emergency departments [27], and even home healthcare [28]. Tools like the IHI instrument may be manual or electronic, but since they require a record review by one or more trained professionals, their use is typically limited to centers with significant resources and dedicated manpower. The tool is designed to detect and quantitate the incidence of predefined adverse events for a given institution.

Automated electronic trigger tools (e-triggers) have also been designed and implemented by a number of large health systems to prospectively surveil for missed opportunities. Routine surveillance can be used to track abnormal tests to ensure patients receive recommended follow-up, and they can be customized to follow and track patterns of error known to be problematic to make sure quality improvement activities yield expected gains [29]. Predefined triggers, checklists, and automated algorithms can identify diagnostic errors in evolution and, in some cases, provide opportunity to correct or mitigate harm. Application of e-triggers can not only surveil, detect, and measure diagnostic quality, but their use can also facilitate institutional learning, guide system design, and provide opportunities to intervene and rescue from avoidable harm.

Patient Experiences and Outcomes

Patients are a valuable source of personal medical information, and they can inform us of common types of diagnostic errors. When patient information is actively solicited from their experience in acute hospital stays, they identify and describe patient safety incidents that are relevant, pose risk, and are potentially preventable [30]. Interviews with inpatients revealed that 27 of 69 patients could recall one or more diagnostic errors during their care over five years for a wide range of conditions and settings [31].

Researchers have learned that patients may communicate about diagnostic error using different language than clinicians, and methods to gather information from patients will be most productive if interviews and surveys are based on an understanding of how patients' reason and communicate about their diagnosis [32–34]. A variety of methods for patient feedback have been studied, including formal patient-reported outcome measures (usually based on functional outcomes), patient experience measures (that capture interactions with providers and the system), and patient complaints and comments (spontaneous or solicited, via electronic or paper survey, or phone) [35]. Techniques to acquire patient feedback include inpatient interviews and surveys;

some have even recruited patient feedback through Facebook [36]. While it is clear that patient reports can inform systems about diagnostic errors, their use varies widely across systems. They provide a useful probe of the system and can add to a multidimensional approach for measurement. It is likely that their role in measuring diagnostic excellence will increase in the coming years.

Formal Clinical Quality Measures Designed for Accountability

The SPADE methodology is well suited to population estimates, and large institutional performance dashboards, and electronic surveillance e-triggers. While patient surveys are useful for local and regional quality improvement, quality measurement for pay-for-performance and value-based care rely on formal clinical quality measures that use robust methods for development that assure they are clinically meaningful, scientifically important, valid, reliable, and generalizable between healthcare sites. The development of formal clinical quality measures useful in national quality reporting is needed to integrate diagnostic excellence as a standard across healthcare systems.

Several barriers have impeded the development of quality measures for diagnosis. There are few good sources of widely available data that have sufficient detail to capture the nuance of diagnostic quality. Administrative and claims databases typically used for quality measure development lack sufficient granularity to be very revealing of diagnostic quality. Measures based on electronic health data are difficult to generalize across different vendors and healthcare sites with varying informatics support. Even though electronic health records (EHRs) have more detail, they still lack structured fields for capturing diagnostic-relevant data. Additionally, standards for diagnostic quality lack benchmarks. These problems helped create inertia that impedes progress, perhaps waiting for improved data infrastructure and interoperability to make measurement easier.

Considerable efforts have been made to advance quality measures for diagnosis by the Gordon and Betty Moore Foundation's five-year investment in diagnostic excellence. Details of that initiative are described in depth in a 2023 listening session with federal agencies [37]. The work supported by the Moore initiative demonstrated that diagnostic quality can be measured with a variety of novel and innovative strategies. Some data challenges can be overcome by linking different data sources. Clinical disease registries can be used to integrate diagnostic information and support quality measures. Proxy measures can be designed to capture relationships that reflect diagnostic reasoning that may not otherwise be documented, such as the use of statins to reflect recognition of vascular risk. Clinical decision support and practice guidelines can be integrated within EHRs to support optimal decision-making while at the same time collecting information about use.

While there is a disproportionate dearth of quality measures that address diagnosis, there are a vast number and variety of processes suitable for measurement. Examples of actual or desired measure concepts suggested by experts in diagnostic safety are provided in Table 12.2 [38–41].

Table 12.2: Examples of diagnostic measure concepts (actual or proposed).

Measure type	Measure concept
Structure	Radiologist services (either in person or remote) are available around the clock for image interp retation.[a,b]
Structure	The institution has a multidisciplinary team available to collaborate on diagnostic cases that are acute, complex, or challenging.[c]
Structure	The organization has an interoperable and certified EHR with embedded clinical decision support.[b]
Process (information gathering)	Percentage of pregnant female patients aged 14 to 50 who present to the emergency department with a chief complaint of abdominal pain or vaginal bleeding who receive a trans-abdominal or trans-vaginal ultrasound to determine pregnancy location.[d]
Process (quality of reporting and communication of test results)	Pathology reports based on lung resection specimens with a diagnosis of primary lung carcinoma that include the pT category, pN category, and, for non-small cell lung cancer, the histologic type.[e]
Process (communication and follow-up)	Percentage of biopsies with a diagnosis of cutaneous basal cell carcinoma and squamous cell carcinoma or melanoma (including in situ disease) in which the pathologist communicates results to the clinician within 7 days from the time when the tissue specimen was received by the pathologist.[f]
Process (appropriate use of evidence)	Percentage of emergency department visits for patients 18 years and older who presented with a minor blunt head trauma who had a head CT for trauma ordered by an emergency care provider who had an indication for a head CT.[g]
Outcome	Patients are informed of their diagnosis.[a]
Outcome (equity)	Diagnosis is equitable between gender, race, and disabilities.[h]

Abbreviations: pT, primary tumor; pN, regional lymph nodes; CT, computed tomography.
[a] Reference [38].
[b] Reference [39].
[c] Reference [40].
[d] Reference [42].
[e] Reference [43].
[f] Reference [44].
[g] Reference [45].
[h] Reference [46].

Priorities and Purposes for Measurement

Measure development and implementation demand resources from healthcare systems that are often limited; thus, judicious choices have to be made to determine priorities for quality measurement. Based on their prevalence and/or their potential for preventable harm, the following areas are priorities for measurement for diagnostic quality improvement:

1. Conditions that suffer the most misdiagnosis-related harm, including three categories (Vascular, Infection, and Cancer) of 15 conditions [47].
2. High-risk settings such as intensive care units and emergency departments.
3. Common problem areas in need of system and process solutions, such as tracking and communicating incidental abnormalities from imaging studies.
4. Disparities and inequities in diagnostic quality.

All measurement is intended to drive improvement; however, measures vary in how consequential performance is for an organization's financial well-being and even their identity. At baseline, measurement priorities are set by regulatory requirements such as clinical quality measures required by CMS or the Joint Commission. While this type of measurement is large scale and involuntary, the targets are subject to public review and typically result from consensus and are driven by the CMS national quality strategy [48]. Measures in national programs are rigorous, require extensive testing for validation, and need to be generalizable and usable across diverse sites. While national programs have few quality measures specific for diagnostic quality, CMS included diagnostic errors as a priority area to make healthcare safer in their Measures Under Consideration (MUC) list for 2023 [49].

Quality measures may be developed and sponsored by medical specialty societies to advocate for new and emerging standards of care that have yet to penetrate healthcare systems. These measures can create awareness and facilitate changes in behavior as well as encourage system design. One example would be quality measures that promote current guidelines for genomic testing for certain cancers, such as the measure for gene mutation testing for metastatic colorectal cancer stewarded by the American Society of Clinical Oncology and included in the Merit-based Incentive Payment System (MIPS) [50].

Measures can also be driven by programs for certification for specialized services, such as the American Heart Association (AHA) Stroke Center Certification or the AHA Lifeline Heart Attack accreditation. These initiatives have been extremely effective at measuring and improving standards of care.

Quality measures can also be incentivized for special recognition by independent bodies. The Leapfrog Group, a private organization representing payors and purchasers of healthcare, publishes hospital grades based on publicly available information. Leapfrog ratings can influence their members' selection of preferred healthcare sites, and a good rating gives the institution respect and credibility. Based on expert consensus, Leapfrog recently published recommended best practices for hospitals that support diagnostic excellence. Many of their recommendations promote basic structure and processes that provide a supportive infrastructure for diagnostic activity [40].

In contrast to national reporting requirements and specialty programs described above, measurement can be highly customized to support specific local quality improvement activities. These efforts can be designed to address high-priority problems identified at the local site. If part of rapid cycle quality improvement, they do not necessarily need rigorous development.

Data Sources to Capture Measurable Elements for Diagnostics Quality

There are many things that are desirable to measure; however, in order to be useful and widely adopted, clinical quality measures must be supported by an appropriate source of data that is relatively easy to retrieve and validate. A variety of data sources are used in quality measurement, but not all are optimal for measuring diagnostic quality (Table 12.3).

- **Manual data abstraction** has been used over time but is a labor-intensive method that is largely outdated now, although it may be useful (or necessary) for selected review of high-risk cases or to investigate cases that are identified by error reports.
- **Claims and administrative data** are the most widely used healthcare data in quality reporting. However, they lack details that are revealing of diagnostic processes and are regarded by many as inadequate as a sole source for meaningful measurement of diagnostic quality.
- **Electronic health records (EHRs)** are a rich source of relevant diagnostic data. Their major limitation is that they are vendor-specific and highly customized. Measures developed with one vendor at one site may not be useful at another without additional informatics expertise and labor. Efforts are advancing rapidly to improve the interoperability of EHRs, and these limitations may be remedied soon.
- **Clinical registries** capture detailed information about specific conditions, and because they are private and designed for a purpose, they can be customized to capture data intentionally to measure aspects of diagnostic quality. Their main limitation is that participation in registries typically requires a membership in the sponsoring organization,

Table 12.3: Sources and characteristics of data for measurement of diagnostic quality.

	Historical approach	Current or novel	Emerging or futuristic
Data type	Largely based on claims and administrative data that have limited value for measurement of diagnostic quality.	EHR and registry data provide more granular details with improved usefulness for diagnosis. Creative data linkages.	Large (perhaps privatized) data sets. Increasing use of AI for automated collection. May incorporate data from wearables and POC testing.
Timeliness of measurement	Delayed, remote from care.	Digitization provides more timely measurement.	Real-time surveillance.
Burden	Labor intensive and costly.	Reduced burden, more automation.	Automatic; though algorithm maintenance will create need for new expertise to monitor and maintain.

Abbreviations: EHR, electronic health record; AI, artificial intelligence; POC, point-of-care.

and access may not be open to all. Like other data forms, they still suffer from the burden required for data collection by participants.

- **Linked data sources** can be cleverly used to better capture meaningful data. One example is novel links between different data sources at various points of care, e.g., pharmacy data with claims data. However, development requires the expertise of a creative and resourceful informatics team.
- **Data from patient wearables and point-of-care testing** are interesting and emerging sources of data; some are finding their way to patient portals through patient-facing apps. They are an as-yet untapped potential source of diagnostic data that could be useful for future quality measures.

Because most healthcare data was not designed with quality measurement in mind, novel approaches to data and analytics might provide interesting solutions. However, to be effective, they will need to be generalizable to ensure that they do not worsen inequities in quality.

Pitfalls in Measurement of Diagnostic Quality and Safety

Measurement for diagnostic quality and improvement has important limitations and consequences, and it is important to recognize pitfalls.

- One can reasonably argue that, in some cases, a failure to establish a timely diagnosis may not necessarily represent an error if a logical rational process was followed and appropriate testing was done. Complex cases and uncertainty mean that we can't expect 100% accuracy on measures for diagnostic quality [51]. A drive to perfection may create other problems with over-testing and overdiagnosis.
- Many actions in healthcare are ideally personalized to patient values and preferences and their unique circumstances, and some of these nuances are difficult to adequately capture in quality measures. Measures should be designed to allow exclusions based on patient values.
- Clinical quality measures can actually erode care if too much emphasis is placed on performance on the measure rather than use of the measure to make the changes necessary to improve. For measurement to improve quality, it must be matched with a commitment to modify the system to accomplish the goal of the measure [52–54].

Digital Measures and the Future of Diagnostic Quality Measurement

While progress has been slower than many hoped, there is good reason to expect acceleration and maturation of diagnostic quality measurement in the near future. Several key advances promise to change the landscape of diagnostic quality measurement: the move to digital quality measures, efforts to define and capture diagnostically rich information in structured fields in EHRs suitable for use in measurement, and the evolving role of artificial intelligence (AI).

CMS has prioritized a transition to digital quality measurement for future quality measures. The 21st Century Cures Act and recent CMS rules have set requirements for healthcare systems to map their EHR to a Fast Healthcare Interoperability Resources Application Programming Interface (FHIR-API) – a policy that will be enforced over time [55]. The eventual result will facilitate the exchange of standardized healthcare data and automatically extract data to calculate digital quality measures. Advancements in digital methods should help move the field forward with more nimble measurement that can allow data to be more widely accessible, aggregated, and used to support a learning health system. Digital measures will likely provide feedback in a more timely way, unlike current methods that often report data long after health events occur. As new digital standards become the norm, it is conceivable that diagnostic data from various sources can be merged, including data from patient portals, patient-reported outcomes, and at-home digital devices.

At the same time, investigators, EHR vendors, and investors are working to define structural elements that better capture data useful for assessing diagnostic quality. The National Quality Forum, in partnership with the American Medical Association, is leading work to establish new standards to routinely code diagnostic data in health records [56]. Demonstration projects have successfully used innovative methods such as natural language processing (NLP) to capture diagnosis information from narrative radiology and pathology reports such that they can be used in quality measures [37, 57]. These efforts aim to ensure that data essential to measuring diagnostic quality are captured and accessible for future diagnostic quality measures.

We are also at a cusp of a technology revolution for AI in healthcare. While many urge caution, the potential for AI to support and improve diagnosis is indisputable. Large language models may improve our ability to capture and synthesize information about patients and even suggest additional areas of inquiry [58]. Prediction analytics may identify and alert clinicians to patient risks. Some potential applications of AI might meld active decision making with electronic capture of compliance with quality parameters such that measurement of diagnostic quality could become routinely embedded in real-time practice and influence care in the moment.

While all these changes also pose risks and need to be developed with caution, it is clear that the future holds many opportunities to measure and improve diagnostic quality [59]. It is not too difficult to imagine a future in which improved access to data and modern analytics provides support for diagnosis while monitoring performance; when it does, measurement may become an automatic process in support of real-time decision-making.

Discussion Questions

12.1 Why have diagnostic errors historically been under-addressed in the realm of patient safety, and how can healthcare systems prioritize addressing this issue?

12.2 The NA framework emphasizes a systems perspective for improving diagnostic quality. How can this perspective influence the development of better diagnostic safety measures?

12.3 How might advances in EHRs, AI, and interoperability contribute to improving diagnostic quality and reducing errors? What challenges might arise from relying on these technologies?

12.4 In what ways can patient-reported experiences and outcomes be better incorporated into the measurement and improvement of diagnostic safety?

12.5 What are the potential unintended consequences of overemphasizing diagnostic performance metrics in healthcare, and how can these be mitigated while still promoting diagnostic safety?

Note: The views expressed in this chapter are those of the author and do not necessarily reflect the official policy or position of the United States government or any agency thereof.

References

1 Saraswathula, A., Merck, S.J., Bai, G. et al. (2023). The volume and cost of quality metric reporting. *JAMA* 329 (21): 1840–1847. https://doi.org/10.1001/jama.2023.7271.

2 National Academies of Sciences, Engineering, and Medicine (2015). *Improving Diagnosis in Health Care*. Washington, DC: The National Academies Press.

3 Leape, L.L., Lawthers, A.G., Brennan, T.A., and Johnson, W.G. (1993). Preventing medical injury. *QRB Qual. Rev. Bull.* 19 (5): 144–149. https://doi.org/10.1016/s0097-5990(16)30608-x.

4 Saber Tehrani, A.S., Lee, H., Mathews, S.C. et al. (2013). 25-Year summary of US malpractice claims for diagnostic errors 1986–2010: an analysis from the National Practitioner Data Bank. *BMJ Qual. Saf.* 22 (8): 672–680. https://doi.org/10.1136/bmjqs-2012-001550.

5 Gupta, A., Snyder, A., Kachalia, A. et al. (2018). Malpractice claims related to diagnostic errors in the hospital. *BMJ Qual. Saf.* 27: https://doi.org/10.1136/bmjqs-2017-006774.

6 Singh, H., Meyer, A.N., and Thomas, E.J. (2014). The frequency of diagnostic errors in outpatient care: estimations from three large observational studies involving US adult populations. *BMJ Qual. Saf.* 23 (9): 727–731. https://doi.org/10.1136/bmjqs-2013-002627.

7 Raffel, K.E., Kantor, M.A., Barish, P. et al. (2020). Prevalence and characterisation of diagnostic error among 7-day all-cause hospital medicine readmissions: a retrospective cohort study. *BMJ Qual. Saf.* 29 (12): 971–979. https://doi.org/10.1136/bmjqs-2020-010896.

8 Wachter, R.M. (2010). Why diagnostic errors don't get any respect–and what can be done about them. *Health Aff (Millwood).* 29 (9): 1605–1610. https://doi.org/10.1377/hlthaff.2009.0513.

9 Graber, M. (2005). Diagnostic errors in medicine: a case of neglect. *Jt. Comm. J. Qual. Patient Saf.* 31 (2): 106–113. https://doi.org/10.1016/s1553-7250(05)31015-4.

10 Reason, J. (1990). *Human Error*. Cambridge, MA: Cambridge University Press.

11 Institute of Medicine (US) Committee on Quality of Health Care in America (2000). Chapter 2. Errors in health care: a leading cause of death and injury. *To Err Is Human: Building a Safer Health System* (ed. L.T. Kohn, J.M. Corrigan, and M.S. Donaldson). Washington, DC: National Academies Press (US), p. 28.

12 Schiff, G.D., Hasan, O., Kim, S. et al. (2009). Diagnostic error in medicine: analysis of 583 physician-reported errors. *Arch. Intern. Med.* 169 (20): 1881–1887. https://doi.org/10.1001/archinternmed.2009.333.

13 Olson, A.P.J., Graber, M.L., and Singh, H. (2018). Tracking progress in improving diagnosis: a framework for defining undesirable diagnostic events. *J. Gen. Intern. Med.* 33 (7): 1187–1191. https://doi.org/10.1007/s11606-018-4304-2.

14 Yang, D., Fineberg, H.V., and Cosby, K. (2021). Diagnostic excellence. *JAMA* 326 (19): 1905–1906. https://doi.org/10.1001/jama.2021.19493.

15 Grob, R., Schlesinger, M., Barre, L.R. et al. (2019). What words convey: the potential for patient narratives to inform quality improvement. *Milbank Q.* 97 (1): 176–227. https://doi.org/10.1111/1468-0009.12374.

16 Liberman, A.L. and Newman-Toker, D.E. (2018). Symptom-disease pair analysis of diagnostic error (SPADE): a conceptual framework and methodological approach for unearthing misdiagnosis-related harms using big data. *BMJ Qual. Saf.* 27 (7): 557–566. https://doi.org/10.1136/bmjqs-2017-007032.

17 Mahajan, P., Basu, T., Pai, C.W. et al. (2020). Factors associated with potentially missed diagnosis of appendicitis in the emergency department. *JAMA Netw. Open* 3 (3): e200612. https://doi.org/10.1001/jamanetworkopen.2020.0612.

18 Vaghani, V., Wei, L., Mushtaq, U. et al. (2021). Validation of an electronic trigger to measure missed diagnosis of stroke in emergency departments. *J. Am. Med. Inform. Assoc.* 28 (10): 2202–2211. https://doi.org/10.1093/jamia/ocab121.

19 Sharp, A.L., Baecker, A., Nassery, N. et al. (2020). Missed acute myocardial infarction in the emergency department-standardizing measurement of misdiagnosis-related harms using the SPADE method. *Diagnosis (Berl)* 8 (2): 177–186. https://doi.org/10.1515/dx-2020-0049.

20 Horberg, M.A., Nassery, N., Rubenstein, K.B. et al. (2021). Rate of sepsis hospitalizations after misdiagnosis in adult emergency department patients: a look-forward analysis with administrative claims data using symptom-disease pair analysis of diagnostic error (SPADE) methodology in an integrated health system. *Diagnosis (Berl).* 8 (4): 479–488. https://doi.org/10.1515/dx-2020-0145.

21 Dhaliwal, G. and Shojania, K.G. (2018). The data of diagnostic error: big, large and small. *BMJ Qual. Saf.* 27 (7): 499–501. https://doi.org/10.1136/bmjqs-2018-007917.

22 The Agency for Healthcare Research and Quality (2021). Common formats for patient safety data collection: diagnostic safety 0.1. *Fed. Regist.* 86 (103): 29263–29264. https://psnet.ahrq.gov/issue/common-formats-patient-safety-data-collection-diagnostic-safety-01 (accessed 25 February 2024).

23 Classen, D.C., Lloyd, R., Provost, L. et al. (2008). Development and evaluation of the institute for healthcare improvement global trigger tool. *J. Patient Saf.* 4 (3): 169–177. https://doi.org/10.1097/PtS.0b013e318183a47.

24 Unbeck, M., Lindemalm, S., Nydert, P. et al. (2014). Validation of triggers and development of a pediatric trigger tool to identify adverse events. *BMC Health Serv. Res.* 14: 655. https://doi.org/10.1186/s12913-014-0655-5.

25 Lipitz-Snyderman, A., Classen, D., Pfister, D. et al. (2017). Performance of a trigger tool for identifying adverse events in oncology. *J. Oncol. Pract.* 13 (3): e223–e230. https://doi.org/10.1200/JOP.2016.016634.

26 Resar, R.K., Rozich, J.D., Simmonds, T., and Haraden, C.R. (2006). A trigger tool to identify adverse events in the intensive care unit. *Jt. Comm. J. Qual. Patient Saf.* 32 (10): 585–590. https://doi.org/10.1016/s1553-7250(06)32076-4.

27 de Almeida, S.M., Romualdo, A., de Abreu, F.A. et al. (2017). Use of a trigger tool to detect adverse drug reactions in an emergency department. *BMC Pharmacol. Toxicol.* 18 (1): 71. https://doi.org/10.1186/s40360-017-0177-y.

28 Lindblad, M., Schildmeijer, K., Nilsson, L. et al. (2018). Development of a trigger tool to identify adverse events and no-harm incidents that affect patients admitted to home healthcare. *BMJ Qual. Saf.* 27 (7): 502–511. https://doi.org/10.1136/bmjqs-2017-006755.

29 Danforth, K.N., Smith, A.E., Loo, R.K. et al. (2014). Electronic clinical surveillance to improve outpatient care: diverse applications within an integrated delivery system. *EGEMS (Wash DC)* 2 (1): 1056. https://doi.org/10.13063/2327-9214.1056.

30 Ward, J.K. and Armitage, G. (2012). Can patients report patient safety incidents in a hospital setting? A systematic review. *BMJ Qual. Saf.* 21 (8): 685–699. https://doi.org/10.1136/bmjqs-2011-000213.

31 Sacco, A.Y., Self, Q.R., Worswick, E.L. et al. (2021). Patients' perspectives of diagnostic error: a qualitative study. *J. Patient Saf.* 17 (8): e1759–e1764. https://doi.org/10.1097/PTS.0000000000000642.

32 Dukhanin, V., McDonald, K.M., Gonzalez, N., and Gleason, K.T. (2024). Patient reasoning: patients' and care partners' perceptions of diagnostic accuracy in emergency care. *Med. Decis. Making* 44 (1): 102–111. https://doi.org/10.1177/0272989X231207829.

33 Schlesinger, M., Grob, R., Gleason, K. et al. (2023). *Patient Experience as a Source for Understanding the Origins, Impact, and Remediation of Diagnostic Errors*, Volume 1: Why Patient Narratives Matter. Rockville, MD: Agency for Healthcare Research and Quality AHRQ Publication No. 23-0040-2-EF.

34 Schlesinger, M., Grob, R., Gleason, K. et al. (2023). *Patient Experience as a Source for Understanding the Origins, Impact, and Remediation of Diagnostic Errors*, Volume 2: Eliciting Patient Narratives. Rockville, MD: Agency for Healthcare Research and Quality AHRQ Publication No. 23-0040-3-EF.

35 Schlesinger, M., Grob, R., and Shaller, D. (2015). Using patient-reported information to improve clinical practice. *Health Serv. Res.* 50 (Suppl 2): 2116–2154. https://doi.org/10.1111/1475-6773.12420.

36 Obadan-Udoh, E., Howard, R., Valmadrid, L.C. et al. (2024). Patients' experiences of dental diagnostic failures: a qualitative study using social media. *J. Patient Saf.* 20: https://doi.org/10.1097/PTS.0000000000001198.

37 The Moore Foundation: CMS Listening Session (2023). https://www.youtube.com/playlist?list=PLopRJPO6GaicIP_7E6rsmgNu4XiraqBQW (accessed 25 February 2024).

38 The National Quality Forum (2017). Improving diagnostic quality and safety final report. https://www.qualityforum.org/Publications/2017/09/Improving_Diagnostic_Quality_and_Safety_Final_Report.aspx (accessed 25 February 2024).

39 Singh, H., Graber, M.L., and Hofer, T.P. (2019). Measures to improve diagnostic safety in clinical practice. *J. Patient Saf.* 15 (4): 311–316. https://doi.org/10.1097/PTS.0000000000000338.

40 The Leapfrog Group (2022). Recognizing excellence in diagnosis: recommended practices for hospitals. https://www.leapfroggroup.org/recognizing-excellence-diagnosis-recommended-practices-hospitals (accessed 23 June 2024).

41 Centers for Medicare and Medicaid Services CMS measures inventory tool (CMIT); Version 1.1. Welcome to the CMS measures inventory tool. https://cmit.cms.gov/cmit/ (accessed 23 June 2024).

42 Centers for Medicare and Medicaid Services CMIT ID: 00734-01-C-MIPS. Ultrasound Determination of Pregnancy Location for Pregnant Patients with Abdominal Pain. https://cmit.cms.gov/cmit/#/MeasureView?variantId=863 &sectionNumber=1 (accessed 25 February 2024).

43 Centers for Medicare and Medicaid Services CMIT ID: 00416-01-C-PQRS. Lung cancer reporting (resection specimens). https://cmit.cms.gov/cmit/#/Measur eView?variantId=1508&sectionNumber=1 (accessed 25 February 2024).

44 Centers for Medicare and Medicaid Services CMIT ID: 00682-01-C-MIPS. Skin cancer: biopsy reporting time - pathologist to clinician. https://cmit.cms.gov/ cmit/#/MeasureView?variantId=2028&sectionNumber=1 (accessed 25 February 2024).

45 Centers for Medicare and Medicaid Services CMIT ID: 00237-01-C-MIPS. Emergency medicine: emergency department utilization of CT for minor blunt head trauma for patients aged 18 years and older. https://cmit.cms.gov/cmit/#/Mea sureView?variantId=1682&sectionNumber=1 (accessed 25 February 2024).

46 Centers for Medicare and Medicaid Services CMIT ID: 01660-02-C-HOQR. Hospital commitment to health equity. https://cmit.cms.gov/cmit/#/Measure View?variantId=13140&sectionNumber=1 (accessed 25 February 2024).

47 Newman-Toker, D.E., Schaffer, A.C., Yu-Moe, C.W. et al. (2019). Serious misdiagnosis-related harms in malpractice claims: the "Big Three" - vascular events, infections, and cancers [published correction appears in Diagnosis (Berl). 2020 May 16; 8(1): 127–128]. *Diagnosis (Berl)* 6 (3): 227–240. https://doi. org/10.1515/dx-2019-0019.

48 The Centers for Medicare and Medicaid Services National quality strategy. https://www.cms.gov/medicare/quality/meaningful-measures-initiative/ cms-quality-strategy (accessed 25 February 2024).

49 Centers for Medicare and Medicaid Services (2023). Measures under consideration list. Program-Specific Measure Needs and Priorities. https://mmshub.cms. gov/sites/default/files/2023-MUC-List-Program-Specific-Measure-Needs- and-Priorities.pdf (accessed 23 June 2024).

50 American Society of Clinical Oncology Merit based incentive payment system measures. https://old-prod.asco.org/practice-patients/quality- measures/measures-library/mips-measures (accessed 26 February 2024).

51 Graber, M., Gordon, R., and Franklin, N. (2002). Reducing diagnostic errors in medicine: what's the goal? *Acad. Med.* 77 (10): 981–992. https://doi. org/10.1097/00001888-200210000-00009.

52 McGlynn, E.A., Adams, J.L., and Kerr, E.A. (2016). The quest to improve quality: measurement is necessary but not sufficient. *JAMA Intern. Med.* 176 (12): 1790–1791. https://doi.org/10.1001/jamainternmed.2016.6233.

53 Rosenbaum, L. (2022). Reassessing quality assessment - the flawed system for fixing a flawed system. *N. Engl. J. Med.* 386 (17): 1663–1667. https://doi. org/10.1056/NEJMms2200976.

54 Kunneman, M., Montori, V.M., and Shah, N.D. (2017). Measurement with a wink. *BMJ Qual. Saf.* 26 (10): 849–851. https://doi.org/10.1136/bmjqs-2017-006814.

55 Centers for Medicare and Medicaid Services (2022). Digital quality measurement strategic roadmap. https://ecqi.healthit.gov/sites/default/files/CMSdQM StrategicRoadmap_032822.pdf (accessed 23 June 2024).

56 National Quality Forum (2024). NQF Partners with AMA to improve diagnostic quality and reduce errors by standardizing patient symptom data. https://www.qualityforum.org/News_And_Resources/Press_Releases/2024/NQF_Partners_With_AMA_to_Improve_Diagnostic_Quality_and_Reduce_Errors_by_Standardizing_Patient_Symptom_Data.aspx (accessed 23 June 2024).

57 The Moore Foundation Transforming healthcare: how groups are working to advance diagnostic excellence through innovative measurement approaches. https://www.moore.org/article-detail?newsUrlName=transforming-health-care-how-groups-are-working-to-advance-diagnostic-excellence-through-innovative-measurement-approaches (accessed 23 June 2024).

58 Adler-Milstein, J., Chen, J.H., and Dhaliwal, G. (2021). Next-generation artificial intelligence for diagnosis: from predicting diagnostic labels to "wayfinding". *JAMA* 326 (24): 2467–2468. https://doi.org/10.1001/jama.2021.22396.

59 Burstin, H. and Cosby, K. (2022). Measuring performance of the diagnostic process. *JAMA* 328 (2): 143–144. https://doi.org/10.1001/jama.2022.10166.

13 Improving Quality Measurement for Rural Settings

Karen Johnson

Quality & Measurement, American Urological Association, Linthicum Heights, MD, USA

Introduction

Approximately 15–20% of the US population – between 44 and 66 million people – live in rural areas (see Figure 13.1) [2]. Compared to their urban counterparts, those living in rural areas have lower per capita income, are more likely to live in poverty, have lower educational attainment, higher unemployment rates, higher rates of food insecurity, higher transportation costs, and a higher percentage of adults over 65 years of age [3–5]. However, some research indicates that those living in rural areas may experience less social isolation than others [6] and have similar feelings regarding optimism about their life [1].

Research also shows that rural residents in the US are relatively less healthy than others, with higher rates of chronic disease, including heart disease, diabetes, chronic obstructive pulmonary disease (COPD), arthritis, and depression [7]. Those living in rural areas also have higher mortality rates overall and for causes such as cancer, COPD, diabetes, heart disease, stroke, suicide, and motor vehicle crashes [4]. On average, rates of obesity, smoking, and methamphetamine use are higher among adults in rural areas, although they are less likely to report binge or heavy drinking [4, 8].

Those living in rural areas often face a lack of access to healthcare, in part due to workforce shortages, geographic isolation, and lack of insurance. For example, compared to other areas, rural areas in the US have relatively fewer primary care, mental healthcare, and dental care professionals (see Table 13.1) [9]. Compared to urban residents, on average, those in rural areas travel further and longer for medical and dental care, and four times as many rural residents as urban residents travel more than 30 miles to obtain healthcare [10]. Finally, rural residents under age 65 also are slightly more likely than their urban counterparts to be uninsured [4].

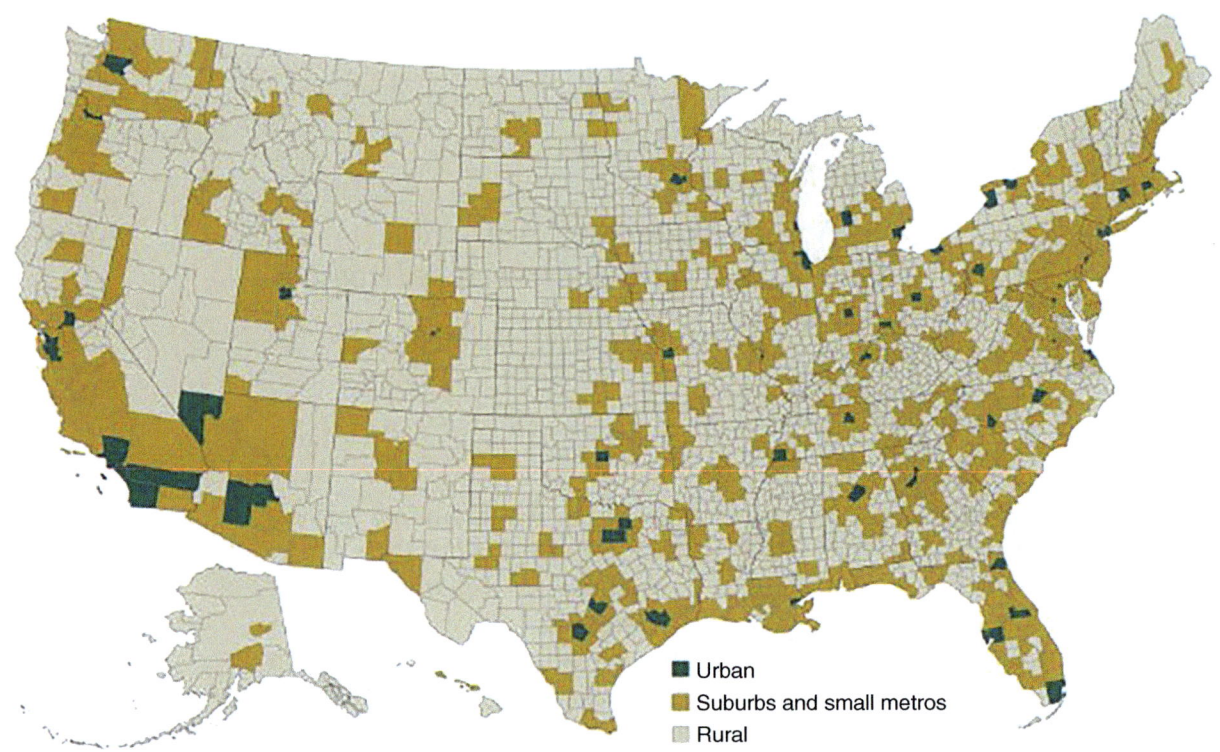

Figure 13.1: Rural, urban, and suburban counties in the US.

Source: Pew Research Center [1].

Table 13.1: Locations of healthcare professional shortage area (HPSA) designations as of 31 December 2023.

Classification	Percentage of HPSA designations		
	Primary medical	**Dental**	**Mental health**
Rural	65.52	66.25	60.38
Non-rural	29.28	28.96	31.93
Partially rural	4.85	4.16	7.49
Unknown	0.35	0.63	0.21

Recent years have seen an increased interest and emphasis in measuring the quality of care in rural settings. This interest has been driven by a variety of factors, including overarching efforts to improve healthcare quality more generally, a focus on inequity in health and healthcare quality and the causal role of social determinants, and the move toward value-based care that relies on results of standardized quality measures. Additionally, there has been a recognition that programs and measures used in current value-based care efforts may not work well for those who practice or live in rural settings.

Recognizing that measurement is a critical tool for improving care quality, this chapter reviews key challenges for healthcare performance measurement for rural settings, describes several best practice approaches that can address these challenges, and identifies future directions for rural-relevant measurement. The ideas presented in this chapter draw heavily from the consensus-based recommendations for measurement in rural settings identified by the National Quality Forum (NQF) in a series of projects funded by the Centers for Medicare & Medicaid Services (CMS) between 2015 and 2022 [11–14].

Key Challenges in Healthcare Performance Measurement for Rural Settings

While not necessarily unique to rural settings, several key issues – many of which are inter-related – complicate healthcare performance measurement for rural settings.

Defining "Rural"

Perhaps surprisingly, there is no one agreed-upon definition of "rural" in the US. Instead, the federal government, states, and other entities define "rural" in various ways to support their own programmatic, regulatory, and research needs [2]. Table 13.2 presents a comparison of three of the most widely used schemas used for defining "rural" in the US.

Table 13.2: Three federal definitions of "Rural" in the US.

Definition and agency	Geographic unit used	What is included in rural	Rural US population	
			Number	**%**
Urban and Rural Areas; US Census Bureau	Census Blocks and Block Groups	All population, housing, and territory not included within an urban area	66,610,922	19.88
Core Based Statistical Areas (Metropolitan, Micropolitan, Noncore); US Office of Management and Budget	County	All nonmetropolitan areas (counties), including micropolitan and noncore counties	46,293,406	14.99
Rural-Urban Commuting Areas (RUCAs); US Department of Agriculture's Economic Research Service	Census Tract, ZIP Code approximation	Primary RUCA codes 4 and above (Micropolitan Area Core, population up to 49,999)	51,112,552	16.55

Source: Adapted from Rural Health Information Hub [2].

The most sparsely populated and/or isolated rural areas in the US are known as "frontier areas." As with "rural," there is no single definition for a frontier area, although defining schemas typically include some combination of population density and distance and/or travel time to an urban area [15]. Depending on the definition used, anywhere between 2.3 million and 12.2 million people reside in frontier areas in the US. Not surprisingly, many of the measurement challenges for rural settings are exacerbated for those in frontier areas.

Fortunately, it is not necessary to use a specific definition for rurality when developing measures or selecting measures for use in specific quality improvement programs. However, the definition can be critical in the implementation phase of measurement, such as when quality measurement programs include special requirements or provisions for those who are considered rural providers (e.g., as in the CMS Merit-Based Incentive Payment Program [16] for clinicians).

Inadequate Risk Adjustment

Risk adjustment in healthcare performance measurement refers to statistical methods that are used to account for patient characteristics when computing performance measures [17]. Such adjustment is needed when patient factors (e.g., clinical, demographic, social, psychological, behavioral, etc.) affect the aspect of care that is being measured (typically, outcomes or cost). For example, if measuring survival after a surgical procedure, older, sicker, or less affluent patients may be more likely than others to die during or shortly after the surgery, even if the care they receive is of high quality. Risk adjustment can help prevent the appearance of worse outcomes for those who care for higher numbers of vulnerable patients when the care provided is of similar quality as that of other clinicians who care for fewer such patients. Without adequate risk adjustment, measure results likely will not correctly reflect actual differences in the quality of care provided (i.e., differences in results may be due to differences in patients rather than differences in care quality).

As indicated earlier, those who live in rural areas often are more disadvantaged than others in terms of their health, sociodemographic factors, health behaviors, and access to care. These factors and others, such as distance to care or challenges in acquiring transportation to care, may differentiate rural residents from others and therefore may impact results of measures that assess the performance of healthcare providers in rural settings. Unfortunately, data for many of these factors often are not available for use in healthcare performance measurement. Moreover, many of these factors may not even be considered in the risk-adjustment process. This may be of particular concern in measurement programs where results for rural providers are compared to those of providers in other settings.

Low Case-Volume

The reliability and validity of healthcare performance measurements may be negatively impacted when too few patients "qualify" for a measure. This "low case-volume" challenge is particularly relevant for rural areas where overall population counts generally are, by definition, low (i.e., because rural areas typically are sparsely populated). Measures with low case-volume are likely to be less reliable, meaning that differences in measure results may be due more to random variation in measurement than to true differences in the quality of care that is provided [12]. In turn, low reliability can invalidate measure results, when those results do not allow for correct conclusions about the quality of care that is provided. Moreover, low case-volume can impact the ability to adequately risk-adjust measures, which will also invalidate measure results. Low case-volume also can impact the reporting of measure results, even if they are reliable and valid, because those results may be suppressed when patient counts are very low to ensure patient privacy. Otherwise, it may be possible to identify individuals and their protected health information (e.g., that they have a specific condition, received certain types of care, or had a specific complication or outcome). The low case-volume problem will be exacerbated when measures target conditions or procedures that are less common overall, which may be of particular concern when measures are being used in an accountability program (e.g., comparison of measure results between providers).

Care Settings with Varied Payment Mechanisms

A substantial amount of healthcare is delivered to rural residents in specially designated outpatient clinics (e.g., Federally Qualified Health Centers and Rural Health Clinics) and hospitals (e.g., Critical Access Hospitals and Rural Emergency Hospitals) [18, 19]. Importantly, CMS uses different mechanisms to pay for care in these settings [18–20]. These payment systems may require use of alternative procedural coding schemas from what is typically used in measures that assess care in other settings or may unintentionally stifle complete and/or precise diagnostic and procedural coding [11]. For example, if paid on a cost basis that is not calculated based on diagnostic acuity and/or where payment is made on a per-visit basis rather than a fee-for-service basis, there may be less incentive to fully document patient problems and provider actions. This can result in incomplete or inaccurate capture of rural patients, their conditions, or their care. In turn, this can invalidate comparisons of measure results between providers, particularly when measures are risk-adjusted. Moreover, those providing care through these settings may not be eligible to participate in certain federal quality improvement or value-based care programs [11]. This impedes the ability to assess, compare, and reward the performance of many rural providers and necessitates the design and implementation of other programs for these settings.

Identifying Appropriate Measures for Rural Settings

A key challenge with any measurement effort is determining what measures should be developed and, if developed, what measures should be used in a particular quality program. As noted earlier, low case-volume, inadequate risk adjustment, concerns with data availability, and differences in payment systems and their attendant sequela may call into question or even "disqualify" certain measures from use in rural settings (e.g., measures targeting less common conditions or procedures or those requiring specialty care). But beyond these considerations, there remains the challenge of identifying measures that are particularly important for rural providers and the patients they serve, given what is known regarding rural residents' health behaviors and outcomes, as well as their lived experience related to social risk and access to care. Identifying meaningful measures for those who live in rural settings is particularly important given that the overarching purpose for measurement is to foster improvement in care for patients and their families.

Best Practice Approaches for Measurement in Rural Settings

Addressing challenges inherent in healthcare performance measurement for rural settings begins with mindfulness on the part of measure developers and implementers of those challenges, along with a willingness to address them to the extent possible. As with the challenges described above, the following best practice approaches for addressing the key challenges in rural measurement are interrelated but are discussed separately for emphasis and clarity.

Consider the Purpose and Design of Measurement Programs

While all healthcare performance measures should be useful for improving access, quality, or cost of care, not all are appropriate for every purpose or program. As such, those implementing measures for a specific program should first consider the level of reliability needed, based on how the program is designed (e.g., comparison against peers versus comparison against a known benchmark) and then consider whether measures that assess rural providers can achieve that level of reliability. They should also "actively anticipate" potential for unintended negative consequences [12] for rural providers based on measure results (e.g., financial penalties that ultimately prevent provision of high-quality care).

Although the principles of good measure design (e.g., supported by clinical evidence, opportunity for improvement, reliability, validity) are purpose-agnostic, measure developers also should consider reliability requirements and the potential negative consequences for rural providers when designing measures for specific programs. Further, to aid implementers in achieving best practices, measure developers also should endeavor to include data from rural providers when developing measures and explicitly evaluate the reliability of their measures for those providers with low case-volume. As part of the development process, developers may need to specify a minimum sample size for their measures to ensure that a reasonable level of reliability is at least theoretically achievable for providers in rural settings. Moreover, they should make reliability estimates transparent so that implementers understand the potential impact of low case-volume (or other limitations) on rural providers who would be assessed by those measures.

Design Measures That Minimize the Low Case-Volume Challenge

Because low case-volume is such a critical challenge for rural measurement, developers should consider designing measures that have the potential to circumvent the problem completely or at least ameliorate it for most rural providers. The 2019 NQF publication that focuses exclusively on the low case-volume challenge for rural measurement [12] identified many such design options, including:

- **Developing Measures That Maximize the Target Population**: This can be done by focusing on clinical topic areas that have broad applicability for all rural residents (e.g., vaccination and medication reconciliation), developing relevant population-based measures (e.g., admission rates for long-term consequences of diabetes), and considering whether exclusions specified in already-existing measures could be modified so that more patients qualify for the measure.
- **Using Non-traditional Measure Calculations That Are more Efficient When Sample Size Is Low:** Many healthcare performance measures are designed to calculate percentages or averages for a certain patient population. However, other more efficient measure calculations should be considered. Examples include ratio measures (e.g., number of bloodstream infections during days in which patients have a central line), continuous measures (e.g., time until medication is administered), and measures that do not have a denominator (e.g., number of infections per month). Use of hierarchical modeling is another example of this idea, although such practice has become more common in recent years and thus may no longer be considered "non-traditional."
- **Finding Ways to Include Additional Patients in the Measure Calculation:** Options for this approach include expanding the

timeframe used in measurement (e.g., two years instead of one), combining data from multiple providers, combining data from multiple settings of care (e.g., surgeries done in both hospitals and outpatient facilities), and using a complex data-driven approach of "borrowing strength" as needed for low-volume providers across time, providers, or other measures (also known as partial-pooling).

Indicate Uncertainty When Reporting Measure Results

As already mentioned, to inform implementers who are selecting measures for use in specific quality programs, measure developers should report detailed reliability estimates as one way of providing valuable insight on how measures perform for rural providers. However, recognizing that no measure is perfect, both developers and implementers should strive for transparency when reporting measure results by also including information regarding the ***uncertainty*** of those results. Possible options (depending on the way the measure is constructed) include reporting numerator and/or denominator counts and confidence intervals alongside measure results. A more recently proposed indicator of uncertainty for healthcare performance measures – one specifically recommended for use by NQF's 2019 rural measurement expert panel – is the exceedance probability [12, 21]. Conceptually, an exceedance probability is the likelihood of being above a certain threshold (e.g., a national average or other useful benchmark). For example, an exceedance probability for a measure result could be phrased as "we can be 84% sure that provider A is performing above the national mean on this measure [12]."

Collect Rural-Relevant Data That Can Be Used for Measurement

The desire for more and better data for healthcare performance measurement is not new, particularly given the focus on health equity and desire by many to account for social risk in measurement. Policymakers and other stakeholders should continue to promote more complete and standardized data collection for such efforts. This could be done at both the patient level and at more of an aggregate (e.g., "community") level [22]. "Rural-relevant" factors – those particularly applicable to rural settings, providers, or residents or of particular important to them – include income, occupation, insurance status, distance and time to care, availability of transportation, literacy levels, and behavioral activities such as smoking.

Consider Rural Relevance in Risk Adjustment

As noted earlier, patient-related factors can impact performance measure results and therefore must be taken into account to ensure that measure results enable correct conclusions about care quality. Accordingly, measure developers should explicitly consider rural-relevant factors when developing risk-adjusted measures. This best practice aligns with NQF guidance to begin the risk adjustment process by building "a robust conceptual model" that "illustrates hypothesized pathways between the social and functional risk factors, patient clinical factors, healthcare processes, and the measured healthcare outcome" and includes at minimum an indicator of urbanicity/rurality [23]. As noted, data for rural-relevant factors that are included in such a conceptual model may not be readily available for use in measurement. Nonetheless, explicitly considering how those factors might interact with other risk factors and how they might influence measured outcomes can help acquaint stakeholders of the strengths and limitations of the measures and inform future development decisions as more data become available, even if ultimately they are not included in the risk-adjustment approach [23].

Develop and Implement Rural-Relevant Measures

As important as the above practices are, rural relevance in measurement should go beyond addressing the low case-volume challenge and adequately adjusting for rural-relevant factors. Also needed is the development and use of measures that address topics of particular importance in rural settings or for rural residents and providers. While acknowledging many of the difficulties and limitations related to both the development and use of such measures, the 2015 NQF Rural Health Committee [11] identified several such rural-relevant topics for which measures are lacking, including:

- Patient handoffs and transitions
- Alcohol/drug treatment
- Telehealth
- Access to and timeliness of care

Assess Care Outside of Rural Settings and Stratify Results

Finally, those interested in rural-relevant measurement should not lose sight of the fact that much of the care received by rural residents is provided by non-rural providers in non-rural settings. Accordingly – *if the goal of measurement is to assess care that is provided to rural residents* – stakeholders cannot focus solely on measurement in rural settings. Instead, they should strive to assess care regardless of geographic setting but stratify results in ways that will best inform improvement efforts for rural residents. Options for stratification will vary depending on what data are available and the number of patients included in a measure. Examples of informative stratification variables include a simple rural/non-rural dichotomy and meaningful categorizations of distance or time traveled for care.

The Future of Healthcare Performance Measurement for Rural Settings

In many ways, the future of healthcare performance measurement for rural settings will follow the same path as quality measurement overall. This includes the development and use of increasingly **more sophisticated measures** – especially risk-adjusted health and patient-reported outcome and experience measures – and the **use of fewer measures** that align more closely to program intent. Examples of the latter include the identification of a core set of rural-relevant measures recommended for use in current or future CMS programs [13] and the move toward use of Merit-based Incentive Payment System (MIPS) Value Pathways (MVPs) in the CMS Quality Payment Program [24].

In addition, the **focus on health equity** in the US will continue, with rurality becoming a more significant subpopulation of interest. This is evidenced by CMS's stated priorities [25] to apply a geographic lens to promote health equity and to increase the collection and standardization of rural-relevant data for the purpose of healthcare improvement. As an example, recent analyses indicate that patterns of care quality in the Medicare population among racial and ethnic subgroups differ depending on their rural/urban status [26].

The use of **telehealth** as a means of increasing access to and improving quality of care in rural settings will expand, particularly once regulatory and reimbursement barriers have been addressed. Although limitations will linger (e.g., imperfect broadband access, deficits in health and in digital literacy), these can be improved. This growth in telehealth as a healthcare delivery modality will necessitate new and innovative measurement. A recent NQF-developed measurement framework focusing on rural telehealth identified five domains for telehealth measurement: access to care and technology; cost, business models, and logistics; patient, caregiver, and provider experience; clinical effectiveness; and equity [14]. As part of this effort, the NQF panel specifically recommended development of new measures that assess the appropriateness of telehealth in specific situations, the comparability of care delivered via telehealth versus in-person visits, and the receipt of appropriate follow-up care.

Advances in **information technology** will influence how healthcare data for rural residents and providers are collected, reported, and used for improvements in health and healthcare. While a full treatment of this topic is well beyond the scope of this chapter, two trends warrant recognition. First is the desire on the part of CMS and others for completely digital measurement. Achieving this goal will require true and comprehensive data system interoperability. While not yet realized, progress continues, as exemplified by the ongoing development, refinement, and use of standards for data elements, data expression, and data exchange. Such efforts promise reductions in data collection and reporting burden on the part of the rural healthcare workforce, as well as near real-time data to support improvement [27]. Second is the rise of machine learning and generative artificial intelligence, the impacts of which are just beginning to emerge. Rural-relevant applications include, but are not limited to, expanded clinical decision support, improvements in diagnostic accuracy, and improvements in healthcare documentation [28], each of which has implications for future measure development and use.

Finally, healthcare performance measurement for rural settings will be strengthened by the implementation of ***value-based care and other innovative delivery arrangements*** that are designed specifically to meet the needs of those in rural settings [29]. By definition, such efforts will require use of appropriate rural-relevant measures and also may drive development of new measures or modifications of existing measures to align with the needs and goals of the programs.

Discussion Questions

13.1 What are the primary challenges in healthcare performance measurement for rural settings, and how do these challenges differ from those faced in urban settings? How might these challenges impact healthcare outcomes?

13.2 How does the absence of adequate risk adjustment for rural-relevant factors (e.g., transportation barriers or socioeconomic factors) impact the fairness and accuracy of healthcare performance measurement in rural areas?

13.3 How does the issue of low case-volume in rural healthcare settings affect the reliability and validity of performance measures? What innovative strategies could be implemented to address this challenge?

13.4 How can quality measurement assess the impact of telehealth for rural patients on access and quality of care?

References

1 Pew Research Center (2018). What unites and divides urban, suburban and rural communities. https://www.pewresearch.org/social-trends/wp-content/uploads/sites/3/2018/05/Pew-Research-Center-Community-Type-Full-Report-FINAL.pdf (accessed 19 December 2024).

2 Rural Health Information Hub (2024). What Is Rural? https://www.ruralhealthinfo.org/topics/what-is-rural (accessed 19 December 2024).

3 U.S. Department of Agriculture State Fact Sheets (2024). https://data.ers.usda.gov/reports.aspx?ID=17854 (accessed 19 December 2024).

4 Randolph, R., Thomas, S., Holmes, M. et al. (2023). *Rural Population Health in the United States: A Chartbook*. The University of North Carolina at Chapel Hill.

5 Day, J.C., Hays, D., and Smith, A. (2016). A glance at the age structure and labor force participation of rural America. https://www.census.gov/newsroom/blogs/random-samplings/2016/12/a_glance_at_the_age.html#:~:text=Rural%20America%20is%20older%20than,participation%2C%20educational%20attainment%20and%20earnings (accessed 19 December 2024).

6 Henning-Smith, C., Moscovice, I., and Kozhimannil, K. (2019). Differences in social isolation and its relationship to health by rurality. *J. Rural Health.* 35 (4): 540–549.

7 Shaw, K.M., Theis, K.A., Self-Brown, S. et al. (2016). Chronic disease disparities by county economic status and metropolitan classification, behavioral risk factor surveillance system, 2013. *Prev. Chronic Dis.* 13 (160088): E119.

8 Rural Health Information Hub (2024). Substance use and misuse in rural areas. https://www.ruralhealthinfo.org/topics/substance-use (accessed 19 December 2024).

9 Health Resources and Services Administration (HRSA) (2024). Designated health professional shortage areas statistics (accessed 19 December 2024).

10 Akinlotan, M., Primm, K., Khodakarami, N. et al. (2021). *Rural-Urban Variations in Travel Burdens for Care: Findings from the 2017 National Household Travel Survey.* Southwest Rural Health Research Center Policy Brief.

11 National Quality Forum (2015). *Performance Measurement for Rural Low-Volume Providers.* Washington, DC: National Quality Forum.

12 National Quality Forum (2019). *Addressing Low Case-Volume in Healthcare Performance Measurement of Rural Providers.* Washington, DC: National Quality Forum.

13 National Quality Forum (2022). *2022 Key Rural Measures: An Updated List of Measures to Advance Rural Health Priorities.* Washington, DC: National Quality Forum.

14 National Quality Forum (2021). *Rural Telehealth and Healthcare System Readiness Measurement Framework.* Washington, DC: National Quality Forum.

15 Rural Health Information Hub (2024). Health and healthcare in frontier areas. https://www.ruralhealthinfo.org/topics/frontier (accessed 19 December 2024).

16 U.S. Centers for Medicare & Medicaid Services (2024). Special statuses. *Quality Payment Program.* https://qpp.cms.gov/mips/special-statuses?py=2024#rural (accessed 19 December 2024).

17 Iezzoni, L. (ed.) (2013). *Risk Adjustment for Measuring Health Care Outcomes.* Chicago, IL: Health Administration Press.

18 Medicare Payment Advisory Commission (MedPAC) (2021). *Report to the Congress: Medicare and the Health Care Delivery System.* Washington, DC.

19 Rural Health Information Hub (2024). Rural emergency hospitals. https://www.ruralhealthinfo.org/topics/rural-emergency-hospitals (accessed 19 December 2024).

20 Medicare Payment Advisory Commission (MedPAC) (2023). Payment basicis: federally qualified health center and rural health clinic payment systems. https://www.medpac.gov/wp-content/uploads/2022/10/MedPAC_Payment_Basics_23_FQHC_FINAL_SEC.pdf (accessed 15 January 2024).

21 Ash, A.S., Fienberg, S.E., Louis, T.A. et al. (2012). *Statistical Issues in Assessing Hospital Performance*. Baltimore, MD: Centers for Medicare and Medicaid Services (CMS).

22 National Quality Forum (2014). *Risk Adjustment for Socioeconomic Status or Other Sociodemographic Factors*. Washington, DC: National Quality Forum.

23 National Quality Forum (2022). *Developing and Testing Risk Adjustment Models for Social and Functional Status-Related Risk Within Healthcare Performance Measurement*. Washington, DC: National Quality Forum.

24 U.S Centers for Medicare & Medicaid Services (2024). Learn about the MVP reporting option. https://qpp.cms.gov/mips/mvps/learn-about-mvp-reporting-option (accessed 19 December 2024).

25 U.S. Centers for Medicare & Medicaid Services (2022). *CMS Framework for Advancing Health Care in Rural, Tribal, and Geographically Isolated Communities*.

26 Martino, S.C., Elliott, M.N., Dembosky, J.W. et al. (2023). *Rural-Urban Disparities in Health Care in Medicare*. Baltimore, MD: CMS Office of Minority Health.

27 U.S. Centers for Mediare & Medicaid Services (2023). dQMs – Digital Quality Measures – about dQMs. https://ecqi.healthit.gov/dqm?qt-tabs_dqm=1 (accessed 19 December 2024).

28 Guo, J. and Li, B. (2018). The application of medical artificial intelligence technology in rural areas of developing countries. *Health Equity.* 2 (1): 174–181.

29 U.S. Centers for Medicare & Medicaid Services (2023). *Advancing Health Equity in Rural, Tribal, and Geographically Isolated Communities: FY 2023 Year in Review*.

14 Implications of Quality Measurement in Workforce Development

Candice Chen

The Fitzhugh Mullan Institute for Health Workforce Equity, George Washington University Milken Institute School of Public Health, Washington, DC, USA

Health Workforce and Healthcare Quality

The health workforce – the people who deliver or support the delivery of healthcare services – is an essential component of healthcare outcomes that affects access, quality, cost, and equity. The characteristics of healthcare workers, their geographic distribution, and whether they provide service to different populations are key drivers of **access to care**. Who is recruited and how healthcare workers are trained, how they are organized, and how they practice impact the **quality and cost of care**, and the intersection of these areas can either advance **health equity** or contribute to disparities (Figure 14.1).

Health Workforce Supply and Distribution

In 2023, an estimated 102 million people in the US lived in Primary Care Health Professional Shortage Areas (HPSAs), while 77 million people lived in Dental Health HPSAs and 166 million people lived in Mental Health HPSAs (Figure 14.2) [1]. The nursing workforce, which had been steadily growing before the COVID-19 pandemic, saw a concerning drop in 2021, particularly among younger nurses whose loss from the workforce will affect health systems for decades to come [2]. During the COVID pandemic, increasing turnover was seen in a number of health professions, including physicians, health aides and assistants, and licensed practical nurses [3].

Health workforce development

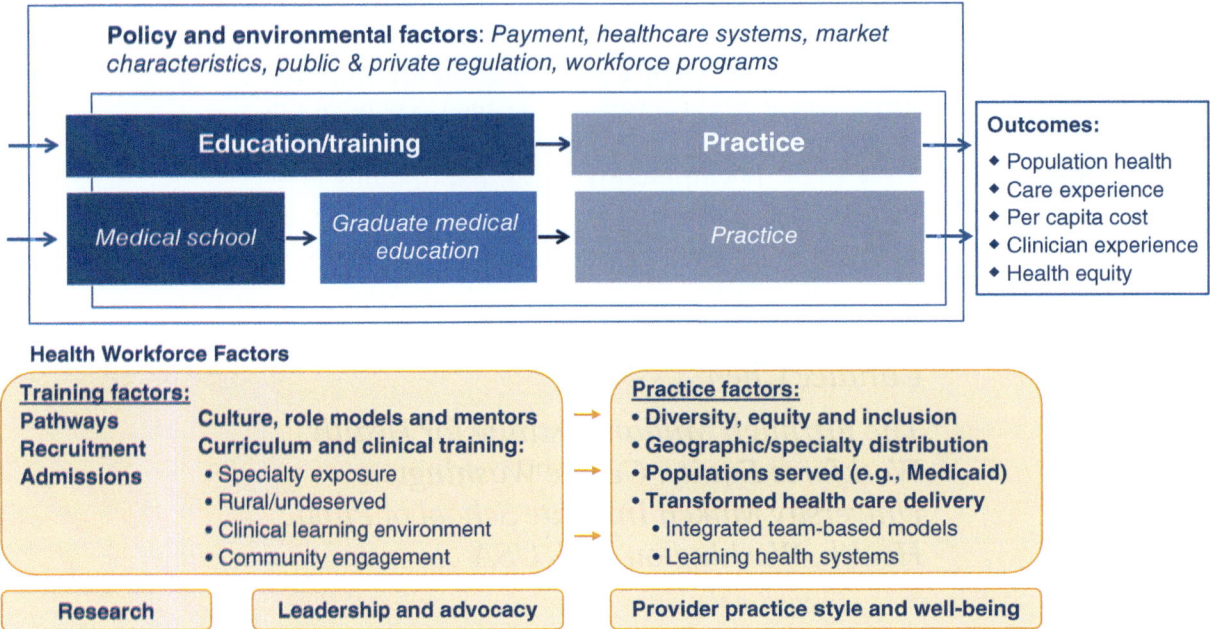

Policy and environmental factors: *Payment, healthcare systems, market characteristics, public & private regulation, workforce programs*

Education/training → **Practice**

Medical school → *Graduate medical education* → *Practice*

Outcomes:
- ◆ Population health
- ◆ Care experience
- ◆ Per capita cost
- ◆ Clinician experience
- ◆ Health equity

Health Workforce Factors

Training factors:
Pathways
Recruitment
Admissions

Culture, role models and mentors
Curriculum and clinical training:
- Specialty exposure
- Rural/undeserved
- Clinical learning environment
- Community engagement

Practice factors:
- Diversity, equity and inclusion
- Geographic/specialty distribution
- Populations served (e.g., Medicaid)
- Transformed health care delivery
  - Integrated team-based models
  - Learning health systems

Research   **Leadership and advocacy**   **Provider practice style and well-being**

Figure 14.1: Health workforce and healthcare quality.

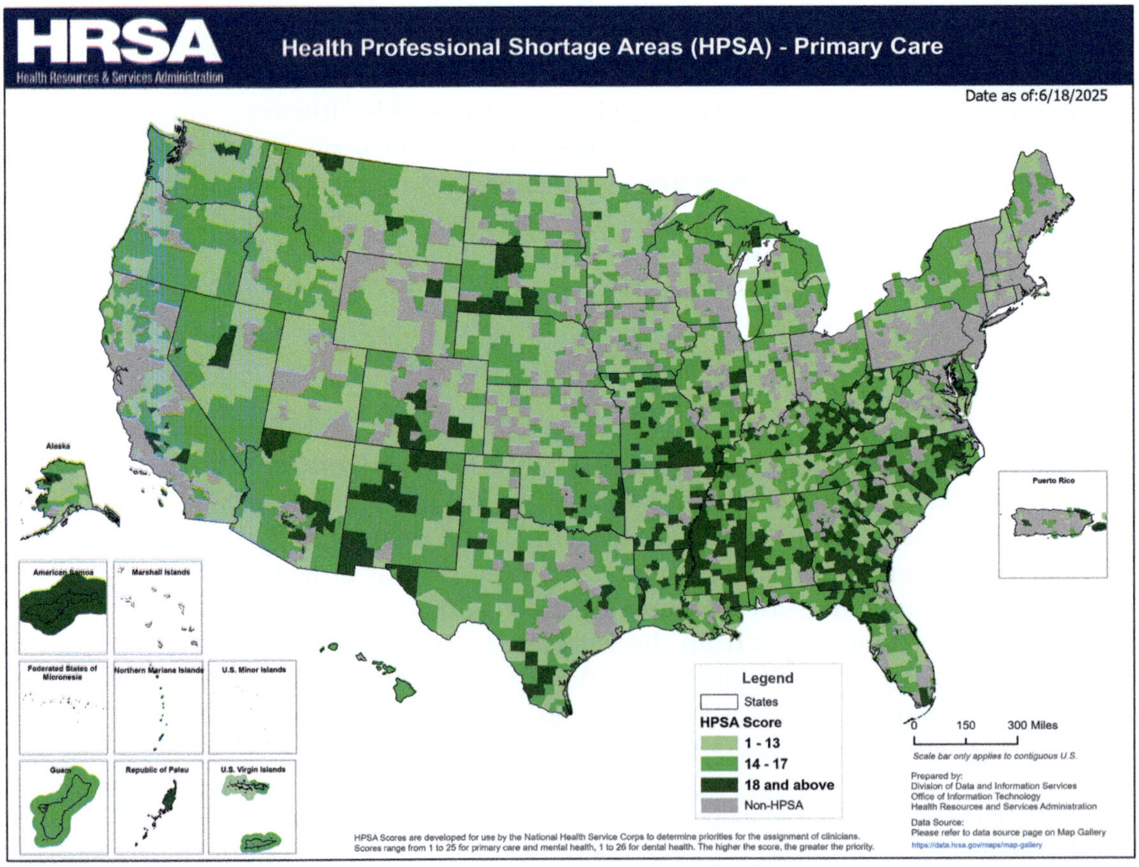

Figure 14.2: Health Professional Shortage Areas. **Health Professional Shortage Areas (HPSAs)** are a federal designation used by programs including the National Health Service Corps, Nurse Corps, CMS HPSA Bonus Payment Program, and the CMS Rural Health Clinic Program for resource distribution.

Source: Health Resources and Services Administration / Public Domain.

Geographic maldistribution of the health workforce is an ongoing challenge for healthcare access. In the 2020 Census, 20% of the US population lived in rural areas [4]. Yet, only 8% of physicians, 11% of dentists, and 8% of psychologists work in rural areas [5], while rural populations face higher maternal mortality, infant mortality, and widening disparities in life expectancy compared to urban communities [6–8]. Urban underserved communities also face barriers related to the health workforce, where the Health Resources and Services Administration (HRSA) projects an adult primary care physician shortage of over 50,000 by 2036 [9], and healthcare providers are less likely to report accepting Medicaid patients, while "secret shopper" studies, where researchers call doctor's offices for appointments, find individuals with Medicaid are less likely to get appointments compared to people with private insurance or Medicare [10, 11].

Staffing, Team Configurations, and New Models of Care

Staffing and the make-up of teams impact health outcomes. In critical care units, higher levels of nursing and physician staffing are associated with lower patient mortality, hospital-acquired infection rates, and costs, as well as better patient satisfaction [12, 13]. Hospital nurse staffing reduces failure-to-rescue and mortality rates and improves burnout and job satisfaction (Box 14.1) [20]. Nursing home staffing levels and instability are associated with quality outcomes [21]. Globally, health systems built on strong primary care have better outcomes [22], and US studies demonstrate Medicare beneficiaries and counties with increased primary care physician supply have better mortality outcomes [23, 24].

How the workforce is configured can also impact healthcare access and quality. Team-based models of care that integrate and optimize advanced practice clinicians, mental health providers, community health workers, patient navigators, care coordinators, and others are showing promise in improving access and outcomes [25]. Innovative models, such as the use of medical scribes, have also been shown to improve the efficiency of care with positive clinician and patient satisfaction [26], and increasing attention is on the role of telehealth and technology to improve access and quality of care, including whether this technology will be equitably available.

Clinician Practice Behaviors

Physicians' practice behaviors can also affect healthcare. Fisher et al.'s seminal work demonstrated large regional variations in Medicare spending that were not associated with improvements in health outcomes [27]. Additional research has explored the supply- and demand-side factors

BOX 14.1   HEALTH WORKFORCE BURNOUT AND MORAL INJURY.

Health worker burnout is a rising issue. Even before COVID-19, clinicians were reporting burnout and intent to leave at high rates, up to 45% and 30%, respectively, in 2019. The pandemic significantly increased the pressure on the health workforce. Early on, they experienced increasing workloads while exposed to a novel, deadly infectious pathogen and insufficient personal protective equipment and resources. Later, they faced ongoing waves of COVID worsened by increasing misinformation that fed distrust and increases in workplace violence. As a result, clinician burnout rates reached 60%, with 40% reporting intent to leave by 2021 [14].

Burnout is defined as a "syndrome conceptualized as resulting from chronic workplace stress that has not been successfully managed," creating feelings of emotional exhaustion, depersonalization, and a sense of ineffectiveness [15]. A related phenomenon is moral injury, which has been defined as "the lasting psychological, biological, spiritual, behavioral, and social impact of perpetrating, failing to prevent, or bearing witness to acts that transgress deeply held moral beliefs and expectations" [16].

Burnout and moral injury result in harm to workers (occupational harms and mental health issues), organizations (staff turnover and increased costs), and ultimately patients (reduced access, patient safety, and quality of care). The drivers of burnout and moral injury in health workers range from relational breakdown (e.g., distrust, values conflict, lack of control, and inequities) to areas of operational strain (e.g., lack of physical and mental health safety, excessive workloads, and inefficient workflows) [17].

National calls to prioritize and address health worker burnout and moral injury have come from the National Academy of Medicine, the US Surgeon General, and other national organizations. Calls for action have all emphasized the need to address the organizational and systems level drivers of burnout, in addition to addressing individual level mental health and resilience [18, 19].

associated with these differences. Demand-side factors include patient health status, preferences, and socioeconomic status. Supply-side factors include healthcare market characteristics as well as clinician beliefs and behaviors. While local healthcare market factors (e.g., financial incentives, availability, and types of healthcare facilities and providers) are important drivers of healthcare utilization and influence how providers practice [28], a 2023 study suggests up to a third of the geographic variation in healthcare utilization can be explained by physicians' practice styles [29].

Evidence further suggests these practice behaviors can be taught. Studies examining the role of residency training programs have shown OB/GYNs' maternal morbidity and mortality outcomes, performance on "appropriate care" questions on Board exams, and spending per Medicare beneficiary can all been tracked back to residency training programs [30–32]. Whether dentists accept Medicaid has also been associated with the characteristics of their dental schools [33].

Health Workforce Diversity

Health workforce diversity is an ongoing challenge with implications for healthcare access and quality. The health workforce faces ongoing under-representation of Black, Hispanic/Latinx, and Native American individuals in higher education and higher income occupations. For example, only 5.7% of physicians and 4.2% of dentists are Black compared to 11.5% of the US labor force. Only 6% of nurse practitioners and 4.4% of pharmacists are Hispanic compared to 18% of the US labor force (Table 14.1) [34].

Students from underrepresented minority, urban underserved, and rural backgrounds are more likely to practice in rural or underserved primary care [35], and an increasing body of evidence suggests the diversity of the workforce (e.g., gender, racial/ethnic, and language concordance) can improve patient outcomes [36–38]. Positive exposure to diverse physicians (African American and LGBTQ) during medical school is associated with less implicit bias [39, 40], and the presence of Black primary care physicians is associated with lower mortality rates for Black individuals at the county level [41]. This early evidence of the value of health workforce diversity is increasingly important in light of a growing literature demonstrating the presence of implicit, explicit, and structural bias in healthcare [42] – ranging from beliefs that Black patients had thicker skin, felt less pain, and needed less pain medication [43] to evidence that Black and Latinx patients are less likely to be admitted to more specialized cardiology units compared to their white counterparts resulting in disparate outcomes [44].

Table 14.1: Diversity of the health workforce.

Occupation	White (%)	Black (%)	Hispanic (%)	Asian (%)
Dentists	67.06	4.22	7.29	21.44
Home health aides	36.66	35.08	21.69	6.58
Medical assistants	50.54	14.65	29.85	4.96
Nurse practitioners	80.17	7.24	6.03	6.56
Pharmacists	66.92	6.32	4.39	22.36
Physicians	64.27	5.74	7.42	22.57
Registered nurses	70.53	11.5	8.14	9.83
Social workers	64.14	20.20	12.05	3.61
US labor force	60.64	11.54	18.02	6.29

Source: Adapted from Ref. [34], https://www.gwhwi.org/diversitytracker.html, last accessed on 28 January 2025.

In considering diversity and equity for the health workforce, it is also important to note that the frontline, lower-income occupations (e.g., direct care workers and medical assistants) are most often women of color. Direct care workers are the personal care aides, nursing assistants, home health aides, etc., who provide service to older adults and people living with disabilities. Over 80% of this workforce are women; an estimated 60% are people of color and 20% are immigrants. In 2021, the median hourly wage for direct care workers was $14.27, and 43% lived in a low-income household (<200% of the federal poverty level) [45]. Yet, this workforce is critical to health systems. During COVID, hospitals reported delays in discharging patients due to nursing home staffing shortages, increasing hospitals' capacity and further straining the hospital workforce [46].

Education and Training

Health professions education and training play a central role in developing a sufficient, well trained, diverse, and equitably distributed workforce. Pathway programs and inclusive admissions policies are important strategies to recruit and diversify the health workforce. Pathway programs provide early exposure to healthcare careers, mentorship, role models, and academic and sometimes financial support and positively impact enrollment in health professions programs, graduation rates, and ultimately practice in primary care and underserved areas [47]. Health professions schools have moved toward holistic review "that takes into consideration applicants' experiences, attributes, and academic metrics, as well as the value an applicant would contribute to learning, practice, and teaching" [48]. Although the 2023 *Students for Fair Admissions Inc. v. Present and Fellows of Harvard College* Supreme Court decision prohibiting the consideration of race in college admissions decisions has created additional challenges for health professions training programs. Prior state "affirmative action bans" have been shown to reduce underrepresented racial and ethnic enrollments across graduate-level programs, including the health professions [49, 50].

Medical school curricula and programs focused on primary care and rural and underserved practice have been shown to increase career choices in primary care and future practice in rural and underserved settings. Similarly, rural training tracks and community health center-based training during graduate medical education (GME) increase retention in primary care and practice in underserved settings [35]. GME, also known as residency training, is the point at which physicians differentiate into the various specialties, and GME in the US is a requirement to become independently licensed in every state. Therefore, GME determines the overall size and specialty distribution of the physician workforce. Evidence also finds a high percentage of family physicians locate near their residency programs [51], suggesting the distribution of GME programs is important for the distribution of the physician workforce.

Health Workforce Policies, Programs, and Measures

The federal government, state and local governments, as well as private professional associations, invest in a number of policies and programs to address the gaps in the health workforce in order to improve access and quality of care. These programs integrate quality measurement in a variety of ways to improve health workforce and patient outcomes. Measures, quality improvement, and accountability are applied at the program and institutional levels, as well as at the individual clinician level.

Federal Health Workforce Development

The federal government *health workforce development* programs include grant programs to improve diversity, strengthen the primary care and oral health workforce, particularly for rural and underserved areas, and expand the nursing and behavioral health workforce; GME payment programs; and scholarship and loan repayment programs in exchange for service in underserved settings, like the National Health Service Corps (Table 14.2).

Table 14.2: Federal health workforce programs.

Name	Brief description
Health Resources and Services Administration (HRSA)	
Health professions training for diversity	Provides grants to health professions schools for the recruitment, training, and retention of underrepresented minority and disadvantaged background students and faculty. Includes the *Centers of Excellence, Scholarships for Disadvantaged Students, and Health Careers Opportunity Program*
Primary care training and enhancement	Provides grants to medical schools, primary care residency programs, and physician assistant programs to support training for future primary care clinicians and faculty and promote primary care practice, particularly in rural and underserved areas
Oral health training programs	Provides grants to increase access to high-quality dental health services in rural and other underserved communities. Includes the *State Oral Health Workforce Improvement Grant Program* to encourage state innovation
Interdisciplinary, community-based linkages	Includes: the *Area Health Education Centers Program*, which provides grants to develop and enhance education and training networks within communities, academic institutions, and community-based organizations; *Geriatrics Programs*, which provide grants to improve healthcare for older adults by developing the health workforce; and the *Behavioral Health Workforce Development Programs*, which provide grants to support the training of behavioral health providers and seek to place these providers in rural and underserved communities

(Continued)

Table 14.2: (Continued)

Name	Brief description
Public health workforce development	Provides grants to support public health training centers and preventive medicine residency programs
Nursing workforce development	Provides grants to support the training of the nursing workforce, including the *Advanced Nursing Education Programs, Nursing Workforce Diversity Program, Nurse Education, Practice, Quality, and Retention Programs, Nurse Faculty Loan Program, and Nurse Corps*
Children's Hospital Graduate Medical Education (GME)	A payment program that supports GME in freestanding children's teaching hospitals
Teaching Health Center GME	A payment program to support new and expanded primary care residency programs made to community-based ambulatory care sites, in contrast to most federal funding for GME, which goes to hospitals
National Health Service Corps	Provides scholarships and loan repayment to primary care clinicians who provide service in Health Professional Shortages Areas (HPSAs)
Centers for Medicare & Medicaid Services (CMS)	
Medicare GME	Payments to teaching hospitals to cover Medicare's share of the costs of a hospital's approved residency programs (largely physician residency programs)
Medicaid GME (federal and state)	Payment largely to teaching hospitals to support residency training programs. Reported by 44 states, payments made through state Medicaid programs are combined federal and state funds

Source: Department of Health and Human Services. Fiscal Year 2024, HRSA Justification of Estimates for Appropriations Committees. https://www.hrsa.gov/about/budget; Henderson TM. Medicaid GME Payments: Results From the 2022 50-State Survey. Washington, DC: AAMC.

While the majority of the health workforce development programs are administered by the HRSA, the largest federal health workforce investment is made through the Centers for Medicare & Medicaid Services (CMS) GME payments to teaching hospitals. In FY 2020, Medicare provided an estimated $16.2 billion in GME payments and in 2022, Medicaid provided nearly $7.4 billion of combined federal and state funds for GME payments [52, 53]. In contrast, HRSA's health workforce programs, which include the grant programs, two GME payment programs, and the National Health Service Corps, totaled $1.8 billion in FY 2023 [54].

Medicare GME has been criticized for its lack of transparency and accountability in meeting the nation's health workforce needs. In 2010, the Medicare Payment Advisory Commission (MedPAC) recommended establishing performance-based GME funding, public reporting around hospitals' GME payments and associated costs, workforce analysis to determine the optimal number and mix of residency positions, and further study of strategies to increase the diversity of the workforce [55]. In 2014, the Institute of Medicine (now National Academy of Medicine) recommended significant reforms, including modernizing payments to "reward performance, ensure accountability, and incentivize innovation in the content and financing of GME" [56].

Research has demonstrated significant variation across programs in GME payments and workforce outcomes such as the production of physicians who practice in rural and underserved settings [57]; however, mandatory metrics and accountability for Medicare and Medicaid payments would require legislative action by Congress [58]. In contrast, the two GME programs administered by HRSA – Children's Hospital GME and the Teaching Health Centers GME – have required reporting by law. Teaching Health Centers are required to report the number and percent of graduates who are retained in primary care and who practice in rural and underserved settings. The Children's Hospital GME program requires reporting on the number of graduates retained in the hospital service areas or within the state. In addition, Children's Hospital GME legislation established a "quality bonus system" to distribute funds based on standards to be established.

State Health Workforce Policies and Programs

State policies play a key role in ensuring *minimum standards* for the health workforce, as health worker licensing and much of regulation occur at the state level. States use licensing requirements to ensure health workers meet minimum standards. In initial licensing, states require minimum training and/or licensing exams, although the actual requirements may vary by state. In license renewals, states often have continuing education requirements that they use to advance different priorities. For example, in response to the opioid crisis, many states required training in the area of controlled substances and substance-use disorders. In addition to establishing minimum standards for licensing, state boards are also responsible for investigating complaints and taking action against clinicians who fail to meet the minimum standards of care. These functions establish an important floor for health worker quality.

These state policies further shape the health workforce in ways that impact access and quality of care. An active area of state policy is scope of practice laws, which determine the services different health professionals can provide and/or the parameters under which they must practice. Scope of practice policies affect a wide range of health professionals, from behavioral health providers, advanced practice nurses, oral health providers, pharmacists, medical assistants, and others. For nurse practitioners, 27 states had unrestricted full practice laws in 2023 (Figure 14.3) [59]. Over time, states with full scope of practice laws have seen an increase in nurse practitioner supply in rural areas and HPSAs [60].

In addition to scope of practice, states are innovating to address health workforce needs. Some states are engaging with nurse staffing laws. California became the first state to require minimum nurse-to-patient ratios

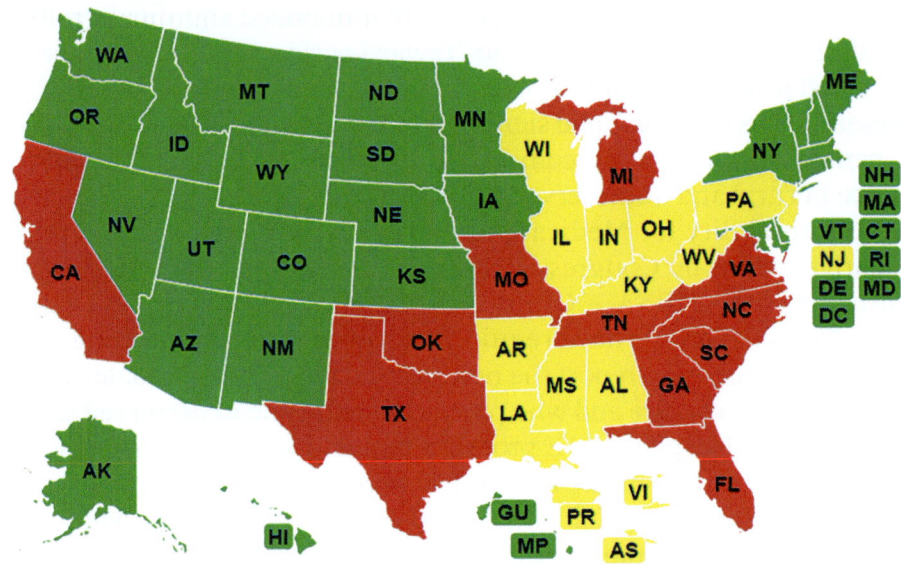

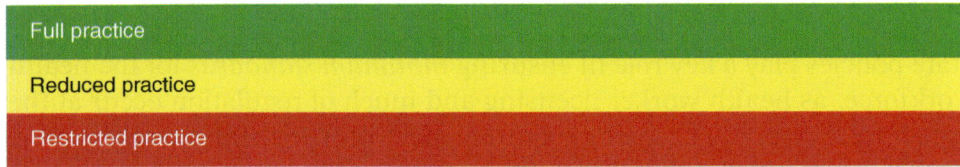

Figure 14.3: State scope of practice laws for nurse practitioners, 2023.

Source: American Association of Nurse Practitioners / State Practice Environment / https://www.aanp.org/advocacy/state/state-practice-environment, last accessed on 28 January 2025.

for hospitals in 1999. Following the passage of the legislation, California hospitals saw an increase in nurse staffing and retention compared to other states [61], and as previously discussed, nurse staffing is linked to better patient outcomes. Minimum nurse staffing ratios effectively establish a structural measure that hospitals must meet.

Similar to the federal government, state and local governments also make investments in the health workforce. These can range from explicit funding to establish new or expand existing training programs, ongoing funding to sustain programs – many health professions training programs exist in publicly funded institutions – and providing grants, scholarships, and loan repayment programs to address specific health workforce needs.

Accreditation and Certification

Professional associations play an important role in establishing *minimum standards* for training programs as well as for individual health workers through private regulation. In the US, institutions of higher education are accredited by non-governmental entities that develop minimum standards and conduct peer evaluations to assess whether those criteria are appropriately met [62]. Accrediting bodies and requirements vary across the health professions. Some professions have multiple accrediting bodies (e.g., the Accreditation Commission for Education in Nursing and the Commission on Collegiate Nursing Education for baccalaureate nursing programs), while others rely on single bodies (e.g., the Accreditation Council for GME for physician residency programs).

Accreditation assures a minimum level of quality of the training program, which ultimately establishes a minimum quality for the graduates of the program. In order to achieve accreditation, training programs must meet minimum standards that address program mission and oversight, sufficiency of educational, faculty, and staff resources, required curriculum and learning experiences, and program outcomes. As an ongoing process, accreditation aims to ensure continuing accountability and maintenance of quality. While accreditation is a voluntary process maintained by private associations, it has been institutionalized through public policies, such as the requirement for accreditation in order for students to receive federal student aid.

Board certification is another voluntary recognition process for individual healthcare professionals. Similar to accreditation, board certification requirements and processes vary across the health professions. Initial certification generally requires individuals meet a minimum training standard (i.e., completion of an accredited training program) and pass a certification exam, and ongoing certification requires renewal.

For physicians, this process evolved to "maintenance of certification" in recognition of the need for continuous learning to ensure evidence-based care in a rapidly changing healthcare environment. Maintenance of certification includes: self-assessment (e.g., ongoing learning and assessment); quality improvement activities; an exam or longitudinal assessment; and maintenance of a valid medical license. The move to maintenance of certification aimed to transition certification from a minimum bar for entry to a lever for lifelong learning and engagement in quality improvement. Although, increased certification requirements received significant pushback from physicians due to concerns of increased burdens and costs [63]. Over time, Board certification requirements have increasingly aligned with other efforts to improve healthcare quality, such as the required improvement activities under the Medicare Merit-Based Incentive Payment System (MIPS).

Health Workforce and Quality Improvement

The federal government has long worked to incentivize and engage clinicians and practices in improving healthcare quality through payment and programs designed to improve healthcare delivery. The *Medicare Access and CHIP Reauthorization Act of 2015 (MACRA)* established the Medicare Quality

Payment Program, combining the prior Physician Quality Reporting System, value-based modifier, and meaningful use programs. The Quality Payment Program is composed of two tracks: the MIPS and the Advanced Alternative Payment Models (Advanced APMs). Clinicians participating in a qualified payment model can participate under the Advanced APMs. Clinicians participating under MIPS receive a Medicare payment adjustment based on four areas: quality, cost, promoting interoperability, and improvement activities (Figure 14.4). See Chapter 11 for more on the Quality Payment Program and alternative payment models.

Numerous public and private initiatives aim to engage clinicians and practices to improve healthcare quality. One example is the Million Hearts® initiative, a national collaborative led by the federal government with state and private partners, to improve evidence-based cardiovascular care. From 2012 to 2016, they engaged more than 500 organizations in a Cardiovascular Disease Risk Reduction Model and in 2017, CMS launched a 10-year Million Hearts® CVD Risk Reduction Model, which provides a payment incentive for organizations to measure and reduce Medicare patients' cardiovascular risks. While the CMS model is ongoing, early evidence suggests participating practices are changing their practice behaviors – increasing their use of CVD medication [64].

<table>
<tr><td>

Quality (30%)

- Report on 6 measures
- CMS will calculate additional measures for groups with 16+ clinicians: unplanned readmissions, unplanned admissions for Multiple Chronic Conditions

</td><td>

Cost (30%)

- CMS calculates cost measures using claims data: Medicare Spending per Beneficiary per clinician, Total per Capita Cost, episode-based measures

</td></tr>
<tr><td>

Promoting interoperability (25%)

- Report on required measures
- Use 2015 Edition certified health records technology
- Conduct an annual security risk analysis and self-assessment

</td><td>

Improvement activities (15%)

- Report 2 high-weighted or 4 medium-weighted improvement activities

</td></tr>
</table>

* Starting in 2023, MIPS also offered MIPS Value Pathways for clinicians and groups to report in a subset of related measures and improvement activities centered around a specialty, condition, or public health priority.

Figure 14.4: Medicare traditional Merit-based Incentive Payment System (MIPS).*

Source: Adapted from Merit-based Incentive Payment System (MIPS), https://www.aafp.org/family-physician/practice-and-career/getting-paid/mips.html, last accessed on 28 January 2025.

Health Workforce Quality Measures

Health workforce measures are also explicitly being used as quality measures. As previously discussed, staffing levels have been associated with quality of care and patient outcomes. The Federal *Nursing Home Reform Act* requires nursing homes to report staffing data to Medicare. Medicare then calculates the ratio of staffing hours per resident day, the percent of nurse staff that stop working at the facility (turnover), and the number of administrators who left the facility, and they report these measures on their Nursing Home Compare site [65]. In April 2024, CMS issued final rules to establish staffing requirements for nursing homes, including, for the first time, a national minimum staffing standard [66].

Medicaid participation is another active area of health workforce measurement. Federal regulations require states to set access standards for Medicaid managed care plans. However, these standards vary widely across states with limited enforcement, and research shows that clinicians listed in provider directories often provide little to no actual service to Medicaid beneficiaries. As a result, individuals with Medicaid continue to face barriers in accessing healthcare [67]. In April 2024, CMS issued final rules to establish national standards for appointment wait times for Medicaid programs and require states to conduct secret shopper surveys to verify Medicaid participation – both are important health workforce measures for access to care for Medicaid beneficiaries [68].

Health workforce measures are also increasingly being used as population measures of access. HPSAs are a type of population measure based on the health workforce. There are three types of HPSAs: (1) primary care; (2) dental health; and (3) mental health. All HPSAs are based on population-to-provider ratios, percent of the population below 100% of the Federal Poverty Level, and travel time to the nearest source of care, as well as population health measures specific to each type of HPSA. HPSA designations are used for the National Health Service Corps, Nurse Corps, Indian Health Service Loan Repayment Program, CMS HPSA Bonus Payment Program, and the CMS Rural Health Clinic Program. In 2022, HRSA established the Maternity Care Target Areas (MCTAs) based on population to maternity care health professional ratio, travel time to the nearest source of care, and other population health indicators for the purposes of providing maternity healthcare assistance to these HPSAs.

States and private organizations are also using health workforce measures to track critical health workforce needs. States like Virginia and Massachusetts have developed "Primary Care Scorecards" that track primary care workforce [69]. Virginia tracks to the county level, identifying counties with insufficient providers [70]. The Milbank Memorial Fund's Primary Care Scorecard tracks state level primary care workforce, including training characteristics (percentage of physicians

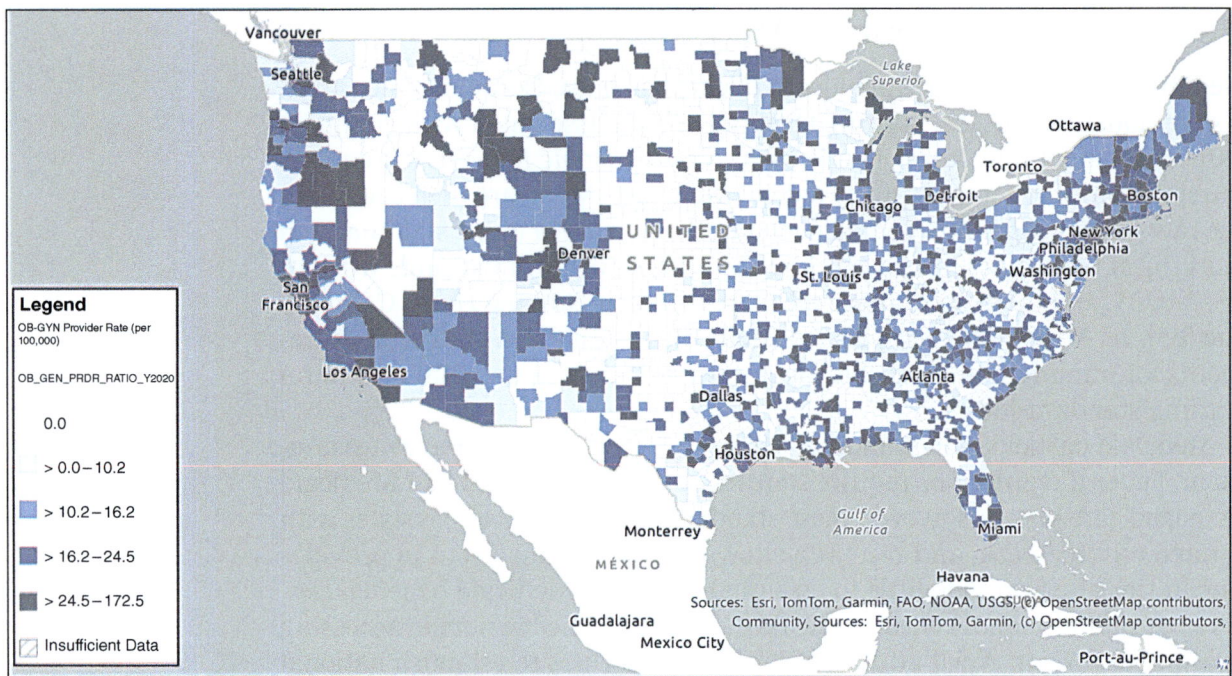

Figure 14.5: OB/GYN workforce.

Source: Maternal and Infant Health Mapping Tool / https://data.hrsa.gov/maps/mchb/, last accessed on 28 January 2025 / Public Domain.

trained in rural or medically underserved areas, medical residents per 100,000 people) [71]. HRSA's Maternal and Infant Health Mapping Tool tracks the potential maternity care workforce down to the county level (Figure 14.5) [72]. These health workforce measures bring clarity to healthcare access and can be used to target policies and programs, track the impact of investments, and further examine the link between health workforce and healthcare quality.

Discussion Questions

14.1 Given the geographic maldistribution of healthcare providers in rural and urban underserved areas, what policies or strategies could be most effective in addressing these disparities? How might these approaches differ between rural and urban settings?

14.2 How does health workforce diversity impact patient outcomes, and what steps can educational institutions and employers take to improve representation of underrepresented groups in healthcare professions?

14.3 What systemic changes could organizations implement to address burnout and moral injury among healthcare workers? How might these changes improve patient outcomes and healthcare quality?

14.4 How can team-based care models and telehealth be leveraged to improve healthcare access and quality in underserved areas? What challenges might arise in implementing these solutions?

14.5 Discuss the role of quality measures (e.g., HPSAs, Medicaid access standards) in improving workforce outcomes. What are the strengths and limitations of using these measures to drive policy and program improvements?

References

1 Data.HRSA.gov. Health workforce shortage areas. https://data.hrsa.gov/topics/health-workforce/shortage-areas (accessed 19 December 2024).

2 Auerbach, D.I., Buerhaus, P.I., Donelan, K., and Steiger, D.O. (2022). A worrisome drop in the number of young nurses. *Health Affair Forefront*. 13. https://doi.org/10.1377/forefront.20220412.311784.

3 Frogner, B.K. and Dill, J.S. (2022). Tracking turnover among health care workers during the COVID-19 pandemic: a cross-sectional study. *JAMA Health Forum*. 3 (4): e220371. https://doi.org/10.1001/jamahealthforum.2022.0371.

4 United States Census Bureau (2020). Census Urban Areas Fact. https://www.census.gov/programs-surveys/geography/guidance/geo-areas/urban-rural/2020-ua-facts.html (accessed 19 December 2024).

5 National Center for Health Workforce Analysis. Distribution of U.S. health care providers residing in rural and urban areas. https://www.ruralhealthinfo.org/assets/1275-5131/rural-urban-workforce-distribution-nchwa-2014.pdf

6 Kozhimannil, K.B., Thao, V., Hung, P. et al. (2016). Association between hospital birth volume and maternal morbidity among low-risk pregnancies in rural, urban, and teaching hospitals in the United States. *Am. J. Perinatol*. 33 (6): 590–599. https://doi.org/10.1055/s-0035-1570380.

7 National Center for Health Statistics (2017). Infant mortality rates in rural and urban areas in the United States, 2014. https://www.cdc.gov/nchs/data/databriefs/db285.pdf

8 Singh, G.K. and Siahpush, M. (2014). Widening rural-urban disparities in life expectancy, U.S., 1969-2009. *Am. J. Prev. Med*. 46 (2): e19–e29. https://doi.org/10.1016/j.amepre.2013.10.017.

9 HRSA. Workforce projections [website]. https://data.hrsa.gov/topics/health-workforce/workforce-projections (accessed 19 December 2024).

10 MACPAC (2021). Physician acceptance of new medicaid patients: findings from the national electronic health records survey. https://www.macpac.gov/publication/physician-acceptance-of-new-medicaid-patients-findings-from-the-national-electronic-health-records-survey/

11 Richards, M.R., Saloner, B., Kenney, G.M. et al. (2016). Availability of new medicaid patient appointments and the role of rural health clinics. *Health Serv. Res*. 51 (2): 570–591. https://doi.org/10.1111/1475-6773.12334.

12 Rae, P.J.L., Pearce, S., Greaves, P.J. et al. (2021). Outcomes sensitive to critical care nurse staffing levels: a systematic review. *Intensive Crit. Care Nurs*. 67: 103110. https://doi.org/10.1016/j.iccn.2021.103110.

13 Wilcox, M.E., Chong, C.A., Niven, D.J. et al. (2013). Do intensivist staffing patterns influence hospital mortality following ICU admission? A systematic review and meta-analyses. *Crit. Care Med.* 41 (10): 2253–2274. https://doi.org/10.1097/CCM.0b013e318292313a.

14 Linzer, M., Jin, J.O., Shah, P. et al. (2022). Trends in clinician burnout with associated mitigating and aggravating factors during the COVID-19 pandemic [published correction appears in JAMA Health Forum. 2023 Feb 3; 4(2):e230002]. *JAMA Health Forum.* 3 (11): e224163. https://doi.org/10.1001/jamahealthforum.2022.4163.

15 World Health Organization (2019). Burn-out an "occupational phenomenon": International classification of diseases. https://www.who.int/news/item/28-05-2019-burn-out-an-occupational-phenomenon-international-classification-of-diseases

16 Litz, B.T., Stein, N., Delaney, E. et al. (2009). Moral injury and moral repair in war veterans: a preliminary model and intervention strategy. *Clin. Psychol. Rev.* 29 (8): 695–706. https://doi.org/10.1016/j.cpr.2009.07.003.

17 The Workplace Change Collaborative at the Fitzhugh Mullan Institute for Health Workforce Equity (2023). National framework for addressing burnout and moral injury in the health and public safety workforce. Workplace Change Collaborative. https://www.wpchange.org/ (accessed 19 December 2024).

18 Committee on Systems Approaches to Improve Patient Care by Supporting Clinician Well-Being, National Academy of Medicine, & National Academies of Sciences, Engineering, and Medicine (2019). *Taking Action Against Clinician Burnout: A Systems Approach to Professional Well-Being.* National Academies Press. https://doi.org/10.17226/25521.

19 U.S. Surgeon General (2022). Addressing health worker burnout. https://www.hhs.gov/surgeongeneral/priorities/health-worker-burnout/index.html (accessed 19 December 2024).

20 Aiken, L.H., Clarke, S.P., Sloane, D.M. et al. (2002). Hospital nurse staffing and patient mortality, nurse burnout, and job dissatisfaction. *JAMA* 288 (16): 1987–1993. https://doi.org/10.1001/jama.288.16.1987.

21 Mukamel, D.B., Saliba, D., Ladd, H., and Konetzka, R.T. (2023). Association of staffing instability with quality of nursing home care. *JAMA Netw. Open* 6 (1): e2250389. https://doi.org/10.1001/jamanetworkopen.2022.50389.

22 Macinko, J., Starfield, B., and Shi, L. (2003). The contribution of primary care systems to health outcomes within Organization for Economic Cooperation and Development (OECD) countries, 1970–1998. *Health Serv. Res.* 38 (3): 831–865. https://doi.org/10.1111/1475-6773.00149.

23 Chang, C.H., Stukel, T.A., Flood, A.B., and Goodman, D.C. (2011). Primary care physician workforce and Medicare beneficiaries' health outcomes [published correction appears in JAMA. 2011 Jul 13;306(2):162]. *JAMA* 305 (20): 2096–2104. https://doi.org/10.1001/jama.2011.665.

24 Basu, S., Berkowitz, S.A., Phillips, R.L. et al. (2019). Association of primary care physician supply with population mortality in the United States, 2005–2015. *JAMA Intern. Med.* 179 (4): 506–514. https://doi.org/10.1001/jamainternmed.2018.7624.

25 Winkelmann, J., Scarpetti, G., Williams, G.A., and Maier, C.B. (2022). *How Can Skill-Mix Innovations Support the Implementation of Integrated Care for People with Chronic Conditions and Multimorbidity?* Copenhagen: WHO Regional Office for Europe.

26 Gottlieb, M., Palter, J., Westrick, J., and Peksa, G.D. (2021). Effect of medical scribes on throughput, revenue, and patient and provider satisfaction: a systematic review and meta-analysis. *Ann. Emerg. Med.* 77 (2): 180–189. https://doi. org/10.1016/j.annemergmed.2020.07.031.

27 Fisher, E.S., Wennberg, D.E., Stukel, T.A. et al. (2003). The implications of regional variations in Medicare spending. Part 2: health outcomes and satisfaction with care. *Ann. Intern. Med.* 138 (4): 288–298. https://doi. org/10.7326/0003-4819-138-4-200302180-00007.

28 Finkelstein, A., Gentzkow, M., and Williams, H. (2016). Sources of geographic variation in health care: evidence from patient migration. *Q. J. Econ.* 131 (4): 1681–1726. https://doi.org/10.1093/qje/qjw023.

29 Badinski, I., Finkelstein, A., Gentzkow, M., and Hull, P. Geographic variation in healthcare utilization: the role of physicians. NBER Worker Paper Series. https://www.nber.org/papers/w31749 (accessed 19 December 2024).

30 Asch, D.A., Nicholson, S., Srinivas, S. et al. (2009). Evaluating obstetrical residency programs using patient outcomes. *JAMA* 302 (12): 1277–1283. https:// doi.org/10.1001/jama.2009.1356.

31 Sirovich, B.E., Lipner, R.S., Johnston, M., and Holmboe, E.S. (2014). The association between residency training and internists' ability to practice conservatively. *JAMA Intern. Med.* 174 (10): 1640–1648. https://doi.org/10.1001/ jamainternmed.2014.3337.

32 Chen, C., Petterson, S., Phillips, R. et al. (2014). Spending patterns in region of residency training and subsequent expenditures for care provided by practicing physicians for Medicare beneficiaries. *JAMA* 312 (22): 2385–2393. https://doi. org/10.1001/jama.2014.15973.

33 Ku, L., Han, X., Chen, C., and Vujicic, M. (2021). The association of dental education with pediatric Medicaid participation. *J. Dent. Educ.* 85 (1): 69–77. https://doi.org/10.1002/jdd.12390.

34 Fitzhugh Mullan Institute for Health Workforce Equity (2023). *Health Workforce Diversity Tracker.* Washington, DC: George Washington University. www.gwhwi. org/diversitytracker.html (accessed 19 December 2024).

35 Goodfellow, A., Ulloa, J.G., Dowling, P.T. et al. (2016). Predictors of primary care physician practice location in underserved urban or rural areas in the United States: a systematic literature review. *Acad. Med.* 91 (9): 1313–1321. https:// doi.org/10.1097/ACM.0000000000001203.

36 Alsan, M., Garrick, O., and Graziani, G. (2019). Does diversity matter for health? Experimental evidence from Oakland. *Am. Econ. Rev.* 109 (12): 4071–4111.

37 Takeshita, J., Wang, S., Loren, A.W. et al. (2020). Association of Racial/Ethnic and Gender Concordance Between Patients and Physicians With Patient Experience Ratings. *JAMA Netw. Open* 3 (11): e2024583. https://doi.org/10.1001/ jamanetworkopen.2020.24583.

38 Diamond, L., Izquierdo, K., Canfield, D. et al. (2019). A systematic review of the impact of patient-physician non-English language concordance on quality of care and outcomes. *J. Gen. Intern. Med.* 34 (8): 1591–1606. https://doi.org/10.1007/s11606-019-04847-5.

39 van Ryn, M., Hardeman, R., Phelan, S.M. et al. (2015). Medical school experiences associated with change in implicit racial bias among 3547 students: a medical student CHANGES study report. *J. Gen. Intern. Med.* 30 (12): 1748–1756. https://doi.org/10.1007/s11606-015-3447-7.

40 Burke, S.E., Dovidio, J.F., Przedworski, J.M. et al. (2015). Do contact and empathy mitigate bias against gay and lesbian people among heterosexual first-year medical students? A report from the medical student CHANGE study. *Acad. Med.* 90 (5): 645–651. https://doi.org/10.1097/ACM.0000000000000661.

41 Snyder, J.E., Upton, R.D., Hassett, T.C. et al. (2023). Black representation in the primary care physician workforce and its association with population life expectancy and mortality rates in the US. *JAMA Netw. Open* 6 (4): e236687. https://doi.org/10.1001/jamanetworkopen.2023.6687.

42 FitzGerald, C. and Hurst, S. (2017). Implicit bias in healthcare professionals: a systematic review. *BMC Med. Ethics* 18 (1): 19. https://doi.org/10.1186/s12910-017-0179-8.

43 Hoffman, K.M., Trawalter, S., Axt, J.R., and Oliver, M.N. (2016). Racial bias in pain assessment and treatment recommendations, and false beliefs about biological differences between blacks and whites. *Proc. Natl. Acad. Sci. USA* 113 (16): 4296–4301. https://doi.org/10.1073/pnas.1516047113.

44 Eberly, L.A., Richterman, A., Beckett, A.G. et al. (2019). Identification of racial inequities in access to specialized inpatient heart failure care at an academic medical center. *Circ. Heart Fail.* 12 (11): e006214. https://doi.org/10.1161/CIRCHEARTFAILURE.119.006214.

45 PIH (2022). Direct Care Workers in the United States: Key Facts 2022. https://www.phinational.org/resource/direct-care-workers-in-the-united-states-key-facts-3/ (accessed 19 December 2024).

46 American Hospital Association (2022). Issue brief: patients and providers faced increasing delays in timely discharges. December. https://www.aha.org/issue-brief/2022-12-05-patients-andproviders-faced-increasing-delays-timely-discharges (accessed 19 December 2024).

47 Rittenhouse, D., Ament, A., Genevro, J., and Contreary, K. (2021). Health workforce strategies for California: a review of the evidence. April. https://www.mathematica.org/publications/health-workforce-strategies-for-california-a-review-of-the-evidence (accessed 19 December 2024).

48 Association of American Medical Colleges. Holistic review [website]. https://www.aamc.org/services/member-capacity-building/holistic-review#:~:text=Holistic%20Review%20considers%20the%20%E2%80%9Cwhole,learning%2C%20practice%2C%20and%20teaching (accessed 19 December 2024).

49 Garces, L.M. (2013). Understanding the impact of affirmative action bans in different graduate fields of study. *Am. Educ. Res. J.* 50 (2): 251–284.

50 Ly, D.P., Essien, U.R., Olenski, A.R., and Jena, A.B. (2022). Affirmative action bans and enrollment of students from underrepresented racial and ethnic groups in U.S. public medical schools. *Ann. Intern. Med.* 175 (6): 873–878. https://doi.org/10.7326/M21-4312.

51 Fagan, E.B., Gibbons, C., Finnegan, S.C. et al. (2015). Family medicine graduate proximity to their site of training: policy options for improving the distribution of primary care access. *Fam. Med.* 47 (2): 124–130.

52 Congressional Research Service (2022). Medicare graduate medical education payments: an overview. September. https://crsreports.congress.gov/product/pdf/IF/IF10960 (accessed 19 December 2024).

53 Henderson, T.M. (2023). *Medicaid Graduate Medical Education Payments: Results From the 2022 50-State Survey.* Washington, DC: AAMC.

54 Department of Health and Human Services. Fiscal Year 2024 Health Resources and Services Administration Justification of Estimates for Appropriations Committees. https://www.hrsa.gov/about/budget.

55 MedPAC (2020). Report to the Congress: Chapter 4: graduate medical education financing: focusing on educational priorities. June. https://www.medpac.gov/wp-content/uploads/import_data/scrape_files/docs/default-source/reports/Jun10_Ch04.pdf (accessed 19 December 2024).

56 Institute of Medicine (IOM) (2014). *Graduate Medical Education that Meets the Nation's Health Needs.* Washington, DC: The National Academies Press.

57 Chen, C., Petterson, S., Phillips, R.L. et al. (2013). Toward graduate medical education (GME) accountability: measuring the outcomes of GME institutions. *Acad. Med.* 88 (9): 1267–1280. https://doi.org/10.1097/ACM.0b013e31829a3ce9.

58 Verma, S. (2020). Letter to The Honorable Charles E. Grassley regarding graduate medical education (GME). January 6. https://www.finance.senate.gov/imo/media/doc/Chairman%20Grassley%20GME%20Response.pdf (accessed 19 December 2024).

59 American Association of Nurse Practitioners. State practice environment [website]. https://www.aanp.org/advocacy/state/state-practice-environment (accessed 19 December 2024).

60 Xue, Y., Kannan, V., Greener, E. et al. (2018). Full scope-of-practice regulation is associated with higher supply of nurse practitioners in rural and primary care health professional shortage counties. *J. Nurs. Regul.* 8 (4): 5–13. https://doi.org/10.1016/S2155-8256(17)30176-X.

61 Mark, B.A., Harless, D.W., Spetz, J. et al. (2013). California's minimum nurse staffing legislation: results from a natural experiment. *Health Serv. Res.* 48 (2pt1): 435–454.

62 U.S. Department of Education. Accreditation in the United States [website]. https://www2.ed.gov/admins/finaid/accred/accreditation.html (accessed 19 December 2024).

63 Teirstein, P.S. (2015). Boarded to death – why maintenance of certification is bad for doctors and patients. *N. Engl. J. Med.* 372 (2): 106–108. https://doi.org/10.1056/NEJMp1407422.

64 Peterson, G.G., Pu, J., Magid, D.J. et al. (2021). Effect of the million hearts cardiovascular disease risk reduction model on initiating and intensifying medications: a prespecified secondary analysis of a randomized clinical trial. *JAMA Cardiol.* 6 (9): 1050–1059. https://doi.org/10.1001/jamacardio.2021.1565.

65 Medicare.gov. Staffing for nursing homes [website]. https://www.medicare.gov/care-compare/resources/nursing-home/staffing (accessed 19 December 2024).

66 CMS.gov (2024). Medicare and medicaid programs: minimum staffing standards for long-term care facilities and Medicaid institutional payment transparency reporting final rule (CMS 3442-F). April 22. https://www.cms.gov/

newsroom/fact-sheets/medicare-and-medicaid-programs-minimum-staffing-standards-long-term-care-facilities-and-medicaid-0 (accessed 22 December 2024).

67 Chen, C., Luo, Q., Bodas, M., et al. (2023). Tracking the elusive Medicaid workforce to improve access. Health Affairs Forefront [blog]. August 2. https://www.healthaffairs.org/content/forefront/tracking-elusive-medicaid-workforce-improve-access (accessed 19 December 2024).

68 U.S. Department of Health and Human Services (2024). Medicaid and children's health insurance program managed care access, finance, and quality final rule (CMS-2439-F). April 22. https://www.cms.gov/newsroom/fact-sheets/medicaid-and-childrens-health-insurance-program-managed-care-access-finance-and-quality-final-rule (accessed 22 December 2024).

69 CHIA. Massachusetts primary care dashboard [website]. https://www.chiamass.gov/massachusetts-primary-care-dashboard/ (accessed 19 December 2024).

70 Virginia Task Force on Primary Care. Virginia primary care scorecard. https://www.vahealthinnovation.org/wp-content/uploads/2023/07/Virginia-Primary-Care-Scorecard-June-2023.pdf (accessed 19 December 2024).

71 Milbank Memorial Fund. The health of US primary care baseline scorecard data dashboard [website]. https://www.milbank.org/primary-care-scorecard/ (accessed 19 December 2024).

72 HRSA. Maternal and infant health mapping tool [website]. https://data.hrsa.gov/maps/mchb/ (accessed 19 December 2024).

IV How Might Quality Measurement in Healthcare Evolve?

15 The Future of Quality Measurement

Helen Burstin[1,2] and Jesse M. Pines[3,4]

[1]Council of Medical Specialty Societies (CMSS), Washington, DC, USA

[2]Department of Medicine, School of Medicine and Health Sciences, The George Washington University, Washington, DC, USA

[3]US Acute Care Solutions, Canton, OH, USA

[4]Department of Emergency Medicine, School of Medicine and Health Sciences, The George Washington University, Washington, DC, USA

Introduction

To envision where quality measurement is going, it is important to consider where it began. Recall from Chapter 1 that early pioneers in quality measurement and improvement included such figures as Florence Nightingale. These individuals showed that systematic action and developing feedback systems for improvement led to measurable improvements in what happened to patients.

For example, Nightingale showed that poor drainage, contaminated water, overcrowding, and bad ventilation contributed to the high death rate of the British Army in India in the 1850s in the Crimean War. She showed that the use of basic sanitation and hygiene standards substantially improved mortality [1]. Another early thought leader was Ernest Codman, a surgeon. Later in the 1910s, Codman conceived and developed the "end result idea," following patients for enough time to know if treatments proved successful and taking measures to prevent new failures when unfavorable outcomes occurred [2].

Quality Measurement in Healthcare, First Edition. Edited by Jesse M. Pines, Helen Burstin, and Jane Hyatt Thorpe.
© 2025 Jesse M. Pines, Helen Burstin, and Jane Hyatt Thorpe.
Published 2025 by John Wiley & Sons Ltd.

Modern quality measurement was originally conceptualized by Avedis Donabedian as three constructs: structure, process, and outcome [3]. This categorization provided an organizational framework for measuring quality into the assessment of attributes of a setting where care is provided (structure), how care is delivered, and whether those services follow best practice or evidence-based guidelines (process) or the results of care and the health status of patients (outcome).

Yet, an issue with the early development of and the now current system of quality measurement is the over-focus on process measures. For example, there are process measures that focus on whether someone received antibiotics for a viral infection when the drugs were not indicated. While it is certainly important that patients do not receive antibiotics when they don't need them, it is not as important as the patients' outcome or Codman's "end result." In the case of infections, that includes whether they recovered as expected, whether their symptoms were optimally controlled, or if they had any adverse effects from any of the treatment. Process measures have been the focus because they are simpler to measure and potentially more amenable to change. Outcome measures are more challenging because it may be difficult to track patients over time and assess whether patients feel better. Additionally, there are many outcomes that are not under the control of a clinician. A patient may suffer bad outcomes despite the best treatment.

Another factor that has impeded the ability to measure quality is that many of the measures rely on data from insurance claims, or what is termed "administrative data." Such information only includes a limited set of data points to use to calculate a quality measure, such as the demographics of the patient, the date the patient was seen, what their diagnosis was, and what procedures or other services were delivered. Since administrative data is often high-level and includes a limited set of data points to use for quality measurement, it has constrained the ability to measure many important, clinically relevant aspects of care. This limits what can be measured and the degree to which selected measures represent the quality of the care delivered.

Other early quality measurement-related efforts included the Healthcare Effectiveness Data and Information Set (HEDIS) in the early 1990s, which measured the quality of care in health plans. Such measures, for example, used claims data to assess whether patients received a specific service in a particular period of time, like a hemoglobin A1C level in diabetics to assess whether blood sugar is under control. In 1999, the National Quality Forum was formed to develop standards for quality measurement, to assemble stakeholders to review quality measures, and to serve as a thought leader in measure development. This set the stage for more rigorous assessment of quality measures, ensured validity and reliability, and broader stakeholder engagement.

Fast forward to the mid-2020s. Indeed, some important changes in the delivery of healthcare and outcomes have resulted directly from quality measurement efforts. One example is the measurement of central line associated bloodstream infections (CLABSI), which occur when patients have large catheters inserted, and the subsequent effort to reduce these infections, which has been shown to be broadly effective in some hospitals. Yet, despite success in specific areas like CLABSI, there is limited evidence that quality measurement has significantly and durably moved the needle on quality nor improved patient outcomes.

There are several reasons for this. First is the dynamic nature and complexity of medical care, which is both highly technical and constantly evolving with new innovations. This makes it difficult to objectively capture some of the discreet actions by clinicians that mean quality care was or wasn't delivered. Second are issues with the data itself, from unstructured data that may appear in physicians' or nurses' notes to structured data from insurance claims or electronic health records (EHRs). Healthcare data is also increasingly complex, located in multiple places, and the same concepts – like whether a patient had a complication or not – may be captured differently in different record-keeping systems. Additionally, some quality concepts, like whether a patient's pain was controlled adequately outside the hospital, may not be measured at all. Risk adjustment can also be a challenge when comparing different patients across settings, with respect to understanding whether the outcomes have more to do with the patient's condition versus the care they received. Another issue is small numbers of patients in a measurement group. For example, a rural hospital may not reliably capture enough information to assess whether high-quality care was or wasn't delivered if there are not enough patients to make a reliable estimate of quality. Finally, when it comes to outcomes, sometimes the goal of medical care may not be uniform across patient groups – like mortality – which may differ based on the patient's functional status. For example, reducing mortality after a severely debilitating stroke may not be what the patient and family want as a goal of care.

Additionally, quality measures have been built into public reporting and value-based payment programs, which reward or penalize providers based on measure results. Yet the measures used in some of these programs have not been sufficiently broad to capture the breadth of clinical and population health. For example, quality measures are frequently process measures that assess a distal step rather than a more important proximal step (e.g., assessing whether a vaccine was ordered or received). More proximal quality measures allow entities to get closer to population level outcomes (e.g., increased vaccination for a given population). Measurement needs to consider other domains beyond clinical quality measurement, including cost of care, patient-reported outcome measures, and equity across patients and populations. Given the focus on the value of healthcare, measures of both cost and quality are required. To avoid unintended consequences, such as stinting to avoid high-cost services, cost measures should only be used in combination with quality measures [4].

To meaningfully move the field forward, the future of quality measurement should address the following issues.

Shifting to Digital Measurement

As technology has advanced, there has been a move from using administrative data to digital data and other sources with substantially more granularity. For example, some clinical data comes from clinical registries developed by specialty societies and others to enable assessment and benchmarking. The widespread use of the American College of Surgeon's National Surgical Quality Improvement Program (NSQIP) provides benchmarked quality indicators for surgical care. Since clinical registries are built by clinicians for clinicians, the measures are often closer to the actionable measures required to drive improvement. NSQIP assesses whether the standard of care has been met for a given procedure, including whether blood transfusions were used, the length of the surgery, the type of anesthesia used, and whether intraoperative antibiotics were used. Using clinical data from EHRs and other sources, clinical registries capture more data points that can be used in quality metrics, including outcome measures, including complication rates. The IRIS Registry of the American Academy of Ophthalmology captures outcome measures across multiple ophthalmic procedures with feedback to clinicians on their benchmarked performance and linked education materials to drive performance improvement.

Recently, quality measures have also moved to gather data from EHRs, which capture detailed data on patient care, including structured data as well as unstructured data. For example, the Centers for Medicare & Medicaid Service (CMS) has an electronic clinical quality measure (eCQM) that uses data from the EHR to assess whether a patient's blood pressure was controlled over a specific time period using blood pressure measurements from EHRs. This is intended to assess the effectiveness of clinician management of blood pressure. Like clinical registries, eCQMs present additional data fields that can be used for measurement, and because they are electronically accessible, they can reduce the burden of human data abstraction.

However, data capture across multiple data sources remains complex, including bringing data together across health systems and even from clinics and from other sources of information like wearables. To advance the field, the clinical community must define the lexicon for measurement, including standardization of core data elements to enable our shift toward digital measures. The use of measures embedded into electronic systems should also be accelerated by the use of advanced technology, including artificial intelligence (AI) and natural language processing (NLP). New requirements that drive toward interoperability will better enable information to be shared in real time across settings of care and will be critical to the future of quality measurement.

In the future, what this may mean is that quality metrics will be drawn directly out of a variety of data sources, including a hospital's EHRs, an insurer's claims data, clinical registries, and other disparate data sources, to create actionable insight. These disparate data sources could allow for important insights, such as delays in necessary care. For example, claims data could be used to track when a test was performed (e.g., mammogram charge), while clinical data could provide test results that suggest that further diagnostic testing is required (e.g., an abnormal mammogram that requires further testing or biopsy). Data from admission, discharge, and transfer (ADT) systems can also allow patient tracking and measurement across settings, such as patient readmission to another hospital. Interoperable data systems provide a more patient-centered view of care, including access to lab and radiology tests from other facilities.

Perhaps the most exciting and revolutionary approaches could be developed with the use of AI. AI can utilize the richness of data in unstructured clinical notes to capture care processes and assess whether evidence-based standards were followed or details on specific outcomes and complications that may not be in unstructured data. AI can also map disparate terminologies – like international classification of disease (ICD) codes, Systematized Nomenclature of Medicine Clinical Terms (SNOMED CT), and Logical Observation Identifiers, Names and Codes (LOINC) codes – to create standardized datasets across systems and streamline the burdens of data abstraction.

AI may also be able to track data in real-time to flag quality issues (e.g., hospital-acquired infections and delayed medication administration). Proactive alerts can also assess important issues like readmission risk, enabling clinicians to intervene earlier. AI also may be able to better account for additional characteristics like social determinants of health, genomic data, and behavioral factors to provide more accurate risk adjustment. Finally, AI may be able to even customize quality measures for individuals, creating adaptive, actionable quality measures tailored to specific populations or conditions – such as patients with rare diseases or with many comorbid conditions.

While all of these would represent a major enhancement in the ability to assess quality from where it is today, successful implementation of AI will require collaboration among clinicians, developers, and policymakers to address technical, ethical, and operational challenges. Yet, with careful design and governance, AI could pave the way for a new era of precision quality measurement in healthcare.

Reducing Measurement Burden

However, in the current system, too many quality measures are used in healthcare simply because they are measurable. A cornerstone of the future of quality measurement should be to stop using measures that do not add value – i.e., they do not drive improvement, they are not actionable, and clinicians and patients do not find the results meaningful. To reduce the burden of quality measures, measurement will increasingly need to be integrated into clinical workflow and digital data sources. This may include the use of AI and other technologies. While measurement of outcomes and patient experience may be burdensome, the future of quality measurement should include a focus on a smaller number of highly meaningful measures at the organizational level, particularly if those metrics are to be tied to payment.

Though measure alignment and harmonization has been a core feature of the quality measurement enterprise, far too many "look alike measures" continue to add burden to clinicians. This lack of alignment also contributes to the epidemic of burnout in medicine. In spite of long-term efforts at measure harmonization, there are persistent issues with similar, though not identical, quality measures across accountability programs (e.g., hypertension control measures that vary by level of acceptable pressure and patient age). AI may be able to harmonize these measures in the long term. However, given the high degree of clinician burnout, often attributed to tasks such as quality measurement, harmonization remains a high-priority area for quality measurement that must be solved in the near term.

Moving toward this goal was proposed in 2023 through the Universal Foundation, a strategic framework introduced by the National Committee for Quality Assurance (NCQA) to improve and streamline quality measurement in healthcare [5]. The aims are to establish a core set of standardized measures that can be applied consistently across various health plans, programs, and care settings to reduce the complexity and burden of quality reporting. Key elements included a core set of measures that address issues such as prevention, chronic disease management, behavioral health, and health equity. Additionally, the framework emphasizes alignment across federal and state programs, health plans, and accreditation processes to avoid duplication and conflicting requirements. It also integrates health equity into its core measures and encourages the use of eCQMs using data from EHRs, claims, and other interoperable health information systems.

Building Equity into Quality Measurement

Historically, measuring equity of care and focusing quality measurement on achieving greater equity have not made up a substantial proportion of the measures in use. While this focus has been increasing in recent years, there is still not an expectation that measurement will always assess and address differences in race, ethnicity, and social drivers across populations. Since some healthcare delivery has a limited impact on outcomes, social drivers of health should be increasingly built into our measurement approach. As data systems improve – in particular, sharing data across disparate sources including healthcare information and non-healthcare information (e.g., housing, subsidized food programs, etc.) – and AI is increasingly used to guide measurement in the future, attention to known inequities in our healthcare system should be routinely built into quality measurement, improvement, and financial performance incentives.

There are multiple approaches to equity measurement, which may play an increasingly central role in quality measurement. As described in this book's chapter on equity (Chapter 9), quality measures can be stratified by population subgroup to assess inequities, provide population level feedback to clinicians, and drive targeted quality improvement efforts. However, stratification may be limited by small population sample sizes and the inability to be sufficiently granular to drive improvement. Direct measures of equity may also emerge, such as the access to and use of trained interpreters, to be directly used to assess and address inequities for marginalized populations.

As social determinants of health are increasingly built into EHR systems, we will have better data to understand the drivers of inequities and develop improvement strategies (e.g., extended hours for on-site pharmacies if adherence is lower in communities without a local pharmacy).

Reflecting the Provision of Care

In the future, quality measurement ideally will increasingly reflect the way care is provided – more team-based care, care across time and setting, and virtual care delivered both synchronously through telemedicine and asynchronously through offline communication. Quality measurement has traditionally been focused on single entities, such as clinicians and hospitals, even though patients are increasingly treated in multidisciplinary teams and fully integrated health systems. The combination of databases across settings and the use of AI may help facilitate this sort of approach.

Meaningful quality measures should increasingly reflect team performance, including quality, equity, and care coordination across longitudinal episodes of care. While some measures, including procedure volume or complications, should still be considered at the level of the individual clinician, many measures, including care coordination and costs, are best suited to assess and support team-based care. While clinicians must be accountable for measures specifically attributable to their performance, the future of measurement should consider how their role is reflected in team-based population health measures. For example, surgical outcomes should logically reflect the entire surgical, anesthesia, and nursing teams, rather than just focusing on the surgeon as the sole driver of care and outcomes. As care is increasingly provided in integrated health systems, teams may also cross settings within systems. For example, infection in a skilled nursing facility may reflect the care of the hospital discharge team, as well as the quality of the care provided in the nursing home. A more comprehensive set of system level measures will drive toward longitudinal measures (e.g., 30–90 day outcome measures) and incentivize communication and care coordination across settings.

The Voice of the Patient

The future of quality measurement will ideally increasingly move to the voice of the patient, including patient-reported outcome measures, patient experience of care, shared decision-making, and care coordination. As the use of smartphones and related devices is increasingly ubiquitous, access to technology should be less of a rate-limiting step going forward. Patient-reported outcomes, including patient function and symptom management, should increasingly be woven into our measurement approach. These results are compelling and useful for both patients and clinicians. Patients should be fully engaged in the co-production of these measures and ensure that what matters to them gets measured. Given the intense need for care coordination in our complex system, newly integrated models of care should incorporate meaningful measures of care coordination, care delays, and missed diagnoses. In the future, measures should reflect the complex handoffs within health systems. Patients can reflect on their own diagnostic trajectories, including missed opportunities for early intervention and repeated testing across settings. Patients can offer a longer reporting lens on complications and long-term function that transcends setting and provider. Patient-reported outcomes, such as patient reports of symptoms and side effects, can not only drive measurement but also have been demonstrated to drive improvement in patient outcomes, including cancer survival [6].

Measurement Science Matters

Measurement science in quality measurement refers to the rigorous application of principles, methods, and tools to develop, implement, and evaluate measures that assess quality, ensuring measures are important, reliable, valid, feasible, and usable. To ensure the appropriate use of quality measures in the future, measurement science must be respected and heeded, particularly with the increased complexity of data and AI. Measurement science issues limit the use of some potentially useful measures, especially outcome measures. This includes areas of concern such as risk adjustment, attribution, threats to reliability and validity, comparability of performance across data sources, and linkage between cost and quality addressed. Shifting the focus from individual measures to a more system of measurement grounded in measurement science will likely lead the field to prioritize interoperable data that incorporate claims, clinical data, and social drivers of care. With more robust data, we can build effective risk adjustment and stratified views that provide population level measurement that can drive targeted improvement strategies, perhaps one day facilitated by AI.

Though the path to digital measures and integration of AI is not clear at this time, the shift to digital measures should enable robust test beds to ensure that reliable and valid measures can be developed and tested with less burden and expense. Finally, measures that can be built on structured fields, coupled with information extracted from unstructured patient notes and narratives using AI and NLP, should move us toward measures of the future that can support accountability and improvement.

Conclusion

Measurement should only be considered a means to achieve improvement and accountability. While measures are essential tools for health system performance, not everything that looks like a nail should be built into our healthcare system to hammer accountability and payment programs. It is critical to be vigilant for the unintended consequences of measurement for both patients and clinicians, such as care stinting and overtreatment only to satisfy a quality measure. The future of measurement should consider Goodhart's law from the field of economics – "when a measure becomes a target, it ceases to be a good measure." To ensure that our healthcare system has the measurement system it needs to improve care, reduce inequities, and incentivize performance, the future of quality measurement must consider and address these issues and how future technologies like AI and others can improve that journey. Quality measurement is a means to an end, and improving patient and population health is the ultimate aim.

Discussion Questions

15.1 What lessons on quality measurement from historical figures like Florence Nightingale and Ernest Codman still remain relevant today, and why?

15.2 Why has there been a historical emphasis on process measures rather than outcome measures in quality measurement? What are the advantages and disadvantages of shifting the focus to outcome measures?

15.3 What are the limitations of using administrative data for quality measurement, and how might digital data sources and AI overcome these limitations in the future?

15.4 How might AI revolutionize quality measurement in healthcare? What are some ethical or operational challenges that need to be addressed to ensure its effective use?

References

1 Kudzma, E.C. (2006). Florence nightingale and healthcare reform. *Nurs. Sci. Q.* 19 (1): 61–64.

2 Donabedian, A. (1989). The end results of health care: Ernest Codman's contribution to quality assessment and beyond. *Milbank Q.* 67 (2): 233–256. discussion 257–267.

3 Donabedian, A. (1988). The quality of care. How can it be assessed? *JAMA* 260 (12): 1743–1748.

4 Ryan, A.M., Tompkins, C.P., and Markovitz, B.H.R. (2016). Linking cost and spending indicators to measure value and efficiency in health care. *Med. Care Res. Rev.* 74 (4): 1077558716650089.

5 Jacobs, D.B., Schreiber, M., Seshamani, M. et al. (2023). Aligning quality measures across CMS – the universal foundation. *N. Engl. J. Med.* 388 (9): 776–779.

6 Basch, E., Schrag, D., Henson, S. et al. (2022). Effect of electronic symptom monitoring on patient-reported outcomes among patients with metastatic cancer: a randomized clinical trial. *JAMA* 327 (24): 2413–2422. https://doi.org/10.1001/jama.2022.9265.

Index

Page locators in **bold** indicate tables. Page locators in *italics* indicate figures. This index uses letter-by-letter alphabetization.

A

Printed and bound by CPI Group (UK) Ltd, Croydon, CR0 4YY

17/12/2025

14794973-0003